*Springer Series on*
# ADULTHOOD and AGING

*Series Editors:*
Lissy F. Jarvik, M.D., Ph.D., and Bernard D. Starr, Ph.D.

*Advisory Board:*
Paul D. Baltes, Ph.D., Jack Botwinick, Ph.D., Carl Eisdorfer, M.D., Ph.D.,
Robert Kastenbaum, Ph.D., Neil G. McCluskey, Ph.D., K. Warner Schaie,
Ph.D., and Nathan W. Shock, Ph.D.

**DAVID A. PETERSON** received his Ph.D. in adult education from the University of Michigan in 1969. His current research interests are the cognitive style of the older learner and gerontological curriculum design. Dr. Peterson is director of and professor at the Leonard Davis School of Gerontology, Ethel Percy Andrus Gerontology Center, University of Southern California. His teaching activities include social gerontology and education in aging.

**CHRISTOPHER R. BOLTON** was granted a Ph.D. in higher education from the University of Oklahoma in 1974. Gerontology education and counseling the elderly are Dr. Bolton's present research interests. He is assistant professor in the gerontology program at the University of Nebraska, Omaha, where his teaching areas include educational gerontology, counseling skills in gerontology, and applied social gerontology.

# GERONTOLOGY INSTRUCTION IN HIGHER EDUCATION

David A. Peterson
Christopher R. Bolton

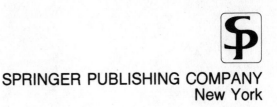

SPRINGER PUBLISHING COMPANY
New York

Springer Publishing Company, Inc.
200 Park Avenue South
New York, N.Y. 10003

80  81  82  83  84  /  10  9  8  7  6  5  4  3  2  1

---

**Library of Congress Cataloging in Publication Data**

Peterson, David Alan, 1937–
    Gerontology instruction in higher education.

    (The Springer series on adulthood and aging; 6)
    Includes bibliographical references and index.
    1. Gerontology—Study and teaching (Higher)—United
States.   I. Bolton, Christopher R., joint author.
II. Title.   III. Series: Springer series on adult-
hood and aging; 6.
HQ1064.U5P47        301.43'5'071173        79-22748
ISBN 0-8261-2860-2
ISBN 0-8261-2861-0 pbk.

---

Printed in the United States of America

# Contents

# 1

# Growth of Interest in Aging and Gerontology

During the past two decades, the subject of older people has piqued the interest and awareness of faculty and administrators of post-secondary educational institutions: Instruction on aging at the associate, bachelors, masters, and doctoral levels has commenced, research has proliferated, and service projects have extended the institutions' resources to local agencies and groups of older citizens. Conferences have burgeoned on numerous campuses, and workshops for professionals and practitioners have become common in all parts of the country. These instructional and research activities have grown slowly, with financial support typically coming from outside the normal resources of the institution. In some colleges and universities, inquiry into various aspects of aging has occurred in several departments simultaneously, and only now are administrators, faculty, and governing boards recognizing the need for increased planning and commitment in this expanding area.

Although awareness of aging in higher education has only recently become widespread, a long history has preceded the current state. These events have primarily occurred outside the field of higher education but are collectively having impact on the traditional disciplines and professions, as well as causing the establishment of new departmental and interdepartmental units in many institutions. A survey of this developmental history will involve a description of demographic changes, social and economic developments, social problems, political activism, and manpower needs of the field of aging. This brief history sets the stage for the involvement of institutions of higher education in the provision of public service, the

1

conduct of basic and applied research, and the conduct of instruction regarding the many phenomena of aging.

## Historical and Demographic Changes

There has always existed in mankind an awareness that the aging process occurs as a prelude to death. Only recently, however, has this knowledge become relevant to individuals. Since people formerly died of disease, hunger, or injuries long before aging affected their physical or mental capacities, the aging process was recognized but its importance was minimal. While long life has always been a goal of human beings, not until the 20th century has it been possible to affect human mortality and extend life expectancy. Throughout recorded history, people have sought magic potions, fountains of youth, and transfers of vitality that would retard or reverse the ravages of time. The search for perpetual youth and extended life are described in the literature of Greece, Rome, and Egypt as well as in stories of the Spanish explorations of the New World.

In 1000 B.C. life expectancy at birth was approximately 18 years (Cutler and Harootyan, 1975). Although a few people lived to old age, most survived only long enough to reach maturity and reproduce before they succumbed to the numerous threats to human life. This condition changed very slowly, for by the year 50 B.C. the average person could anticipate only 25 years of life. It was not until the year 1600 A.D. that life expectancy reached 32 years, and by the beginning of the 20th century, the average individual lived to only 49 years (Siegel, 1976). The early part of the 20th century saw a rapid growth in life expectancy. By 1939 the individual could expect to live until age 63, a 16 year increase in four decades (Cutler and Harootyan, 1975). This extension resulted from our nation's growing understanding and promotion of public health as well as control of communicable diseases such as smallpox, diphtheria, typhoid, and TB. Today, life expectancy of a female at birth is 75 years, while males can anticipate 68 years of life (Woodruff, 1975). Thus, most of us will experience old age and determine for ourselves whether the added years which have been sought for centuries are a reward or a curse.

This lengthened life expectancy has resulted in a major growth of the older population. In 1974 there were 22 million persons over the age of 65—approximately 10 percent of the total U.S. population (Siegel, 1976). By the year 2000 the total is expected to be 30 million, an additional 10 million persons will be between the ages of 60 and

65, and this group will be increasing by over 400,000 annually. That will mean that 11.7 percent of the population will then be age 65+ and 15.5 percent will be over age 60 (Siegel, 1976).

The number and percent of older persons in the U.S. are expected to peak between 2010 and 2025 when the cohort of the post-World War II baby boom reaches age 65. Until that time, it is reasonable to expect that there will continue to be a growing awareness of the needs of this group and appropriate responses on the part of many social institutions. If additional breakthroughs occur in medical science so that cancer, heart disease, or stroke is controlled or eliminated, the number of older people will grow even faster and the needs of an aging society will be accelerated.

According to Rockstein and his colleagues (1977), the average human being has a potential life span of approximately 110 to 115 years, yet the majority of us do not live that long because we have not prevented the insults and illnesses that shorten life. We die, not from old age, but from the accompaniments of modern life such as stress, obesity, sedentariness, smoking, and automobile accidents. If some of those accompaniments were to be controlled more satisfactorily by medical science or if public education were able to convince us to live in a healthful way, the results could be a significant extension of life for the average American.

## Social Impact of the Aging Cohort

The effects of an expanding older population are increasingly evident in the social, economic, and political structure of our society. As the size of the aged population increases, older individuals tend to decline in status because they are no longer scarce and seldom provide a unique contribution to modern society. Their role as carriers of culture and history has been replaced by educational institutions and the media, which provide understanding of the past and knowledge of the present; they no longer serve as the link with former generations. Rather, their role becomes unclear and their value to society becomes open to question.

Perhaps the greatest change in roles comes in the increasing proportion of older persons who are no longer employed. In 1900 only one-third of the 65+ population was retired; today over 75 percent of this group is outside the work force (Siegel, 1976). The economic, social, and psychological influence of retirement, a new phenomenon, on the older population is pervasive. Although many older people adjust quickly and easily to a life filled with leisure, others find that their self-view is closely tied to their occupational role, and when that is removed, they have difficulty maintaining their self-image, self-esteem, and self-motivation.

The economic cost of maintaining millions of adults outside the work force is enormous. A major portion of this cost is borne by the federal government, which will spend over $100 billion, nearly one-fourth of the total federal budget, on programs and services for the elderly during 1977–78 (Powell, 1979). Moreover, the full cost of this commitment must take into account the additional billions allocated by states, local governments, and voluntary and private agencies for programs for the older population. These include not only the income maintenance programs of social security and supplementary security income, but health insurance, housing, social services, transportation, nutrition, recreation, education, and government pensions.

The economic implications of an aging population are not limited to government and voluntary programs in the social and health fields. Public and private pension funds now own over one-third of all equities (stock) of American business and industry. This ownership may be expected to continue growing in the future and by 1985 will include over half of all stock and a major portion of all debt capital (bonds, debentures, and notes) (Drucker, 1976). If retirees are hurt in the future by increased inflation and taxes, they may force pension administrators to pressure corporations into paying additional dividends in order to increase their income. As a result, corporations could have less capital to reinvest in plant and equipment, a condition that could lead to slowed economic growth.

The commitment by the federal government to provide a decent standard of living for older persons has coincided with media and social reform chronicles of the difficulties of the old. Just as the Great Society programs of the 1960s brought to light the problems of minorities and the poor, so the aged are now becoming increasingly visible and demanding their share of the national wealth. They are choosing to use the political process in order to make their situation known and to secure increased support for income maintenance, health, and community service programs.

Over the past decade, social programs for minorities and the poor have been created and quickly subsided. The continuation and expansion of aging programs may be explained by our conviction that since older persons have contributed to the welfare of this country for many years, they do not deserve to suffer in later life. Furthermore, each of us is aware of our own aging: We realize that by establishing systems that care for the current elderly, we are assuring that our own later years will be pleasant and relatively worry free.

We are beginning to glimpse the outline of a future America substantially modified by the growth of the older population. The financial support to this group, new roles and meanings for longer life, social and health needs as well as new and innovative approaches, and the general awareness of the accompaniments of an aging society will all increase. It is very possible that conflicts between the working and retired populations over use of resources will escalate. The outcome is not clear at this time, but the future will witness substantial changes as the result of an aging society.

## Elements of Social Activism

The past 20 years have seen a growing emphasis on community programs and services for the aging. This focus has become so strong that it is assuming many of the characteristics of a social movement. Activist philosophy is currently at a high level, and community organizers, older people, and academics are combining forces to attack the societal inadequacies detrimental to older people. However, recently these problems have come to be perceived as so large and pervasive that the family, voluntary agencies, or philanthropic organizations cannot adequately address them. Only government resources can provide the needed financial base.

Advocates for the aging now recognize that the key to expanded social programs lies in the ability of older people to demand and receive financial aid from Washington. The aging coalition has found that it can deal more effectively with the members of the federal Congress and the staffs of the numerous committees than it can with state and local politicians and competing groups. Consequently, the current emphasis of much aging activity is to persuade Representatives and Senators that the needs of older people are extensive and unmet.

There are several advocate groups, developed over the past 20 years, that are composed primarily of older people. The American Association of Retired Persons/National Retired Teacher's Association claims over 11 million dues-paying members past the age of 55; the National Council of Senior Citizens and the Grey Panthers, though not as large as AARP/NRTA, have political action as their primary interest, with most of their members committed to this approach.

These groups work closely with the staff and membership of several Congressional Committees with a major interest in aging-related legislation. The Senate Special Committee on Aging and the House Select Committee on Aging, although not authorized to introduce legislation, take an active role in advocacy within Congress on behalf of older people. Senior citizen organizations have also found a ready ally in bureaucrats who administer programs for the aging. Within the federal government, the Administration on Aging, the National Institute on Aging, the Social Security Administration, the Health Services Administration, and the Public Health Service all have staff members who have interest in older citizens and support the continuation and expansion of current programs.

The White House Conferences on Aging held in 1961 and 1971 encouraged the growing awareness of older persons' needs and the development of organizations and agencies collectively supporting age-related programs. These national meetings of consumers, politicians, and agency representatives have drawn the attention of policy makers and federal administrative personnel, as well as the public, to the current situation of older persons. Each White House Conference proved to be a major motivation for programs and legislation for the aging.

College and university faculty have not been isolated from these political and community developments. Although interest in aging may have begun as a scholarly pursuit, it is not uncommon to find faculty heavily involved in the planning and operation of local programs, in the development of strategy for expanding funding and legislative mandates, or in the consciousness raising that is necessary for the continuation of these programs. Thus, educators, community leaders, bureaucrats, politicians, and the aging themselves have joined together to identify needs, seek funds, and operate programs that can replace the support systems traditionally provided by the family for the few who lived to be old.

## Manpower Preparation for the Field of Aging

The expansion of federally and locally funded programs for older people has opened major opportunities for employment, often appropriate to persons holding the bachelor's or master's degree. At a time when some traditional employment markets for college graduates have begun to contract, the opportunities in local, state, and federal programs serving older people have attracted the attention of both faculty and students. Services to older people require increasing numbers of personnel who have an understanding of the developmental processes of aging, an interest in working with this client group, and an understanding of the service delivery structure now emerging. Since service to older people is a labor-intensive undertaking, the potential opportunities are immense, and increased attention is being devoted to preparing individuals for current and future positions.

Colleges and universities have responded to this situation by designing courses and curricula to help students gain an understanding of gerontology as well as prepare them for available positions. These programs have a variety of foci, but generally emphasize (1) sensitization of the student to the older population; (2) acquisition of accurate knowledge about the older person; (3) understanding of the social accompaniments of growing old in this society; (4) dealing with students' own feelings about old age, dependency, and death; (5) awareness of the network of agencies providing services to older people; and (6) development of skills that will be salable to these agencies.

Most of the courses of study combine two or more of these foci in a manner that provides the student with some of the skills needed for employment. This is often supplemented with a semester or two of field work, which offers the opportunity to utilize some of the skills acquired in the classroom and to experience firsthand the operation of a community agency or institution.

Numerous community colleges have begun to offer courses on working with older people. Persons trained at the aide or technician level typically find jobs in institutions such as nursing homes, hospitals, homes for the aged, or state mental institutions or in community settings as home health aides, homemakers, handymen, or companions. Although this instruction is both needed and useful, salaries do not always reflect the additional preparation. Many of these positions are currently filled by staff with little or no formal training, and there is limited indication of a market that will use or pay personnel adequately in the immediate future.

Positions for college graduates vary significantly by profession and region. Even with inconsistencies, however, there are some patterns emerging. Direct service jobs for persons at the bachelor's level include recreation, social services, nursing, administration, outreach, counseling, information and referral, and program planning. In most cases the employee is likely to have direct contact with older clients as well as have the opportunity to supervise the work of paraprofessionals and/or volunteers. Persons who have completed a master's degree are more likely to find positions available at the planning, evaluation, administration, instruction, or supervisory level in institutions and community programs. These may be nurses, administrators in area agencies on aging, personnel in state offices on aging, social workers, nutritionists, recreation coordinators, counselors, clinicians, evaluators, or program planners. In general, the larger metropolitan areas are more likely to have positions and salaries for persons with the higher levels of education, and many graduates find it necessary to move to those areas.

Positions for persons who have completed a doctorate and are interested in the area of aging are becoming more common. Colleges and universities expanding their instructional programs in gerontology seek such persons, as do research centers concerned with the phenomena of aging. Institutions of higher education and other organizations are finding much demand for continuing education of practitioners and are seeking well qualified persons to prepare and conduct these workshops, seminars, and short training sessions. Several consulting firms as well as many universities are heavily involved in project evaluation and the development of service delivery models for community programs. The federal government is also a major employer of persons prepared at the doctoral level and may be expected to intensify recruitment as the field becomes more sophisticated, thereby creating a need for personnel who are skilled in research and program management. The increased elderly population is exerting pressure on the federal government for more services. It is reasonable to assume that as more programs and trained personnel become available, the aging will respond with expanded use of service.

As time passes, it is probable that more and more of the personnel who work in the field of aging will hold advanced degrees and that they will be expected to have some specific preparation in gerontology. Although it is not completely clear how soon or in what manner this will be implemented, there is a discernible trend toward professionalization of the field and a desire to assure that some gerontological knowledge is included along with technical skills. Thus, the future is likely to hold more gerontology instruction, an event which will require institutions of higher education to expand their offerings in this area.

## Conclusion

The increased visibility of the aging is concurrent with changes in life expectancy, the growth of the older population, the perceived needs of this group, and the availability of program funding to alleviate their social and health needs. Institutions of higher education have become involved through advocacy for expanded programs, planning and evaluation of these services, and preparation of students who will carry out the legislative mandate to improve the quality of life of older Americans. Research, technical assistance, continuing education, and community service activities have quickly followed as increasingly larger numbers of educational institutions have realized the potential that the field of aging holds.

For a time it was popular to question the reasons why there were so few higher education programs in the gerontological area. Now there is so much activity that the questions are shifting to the quality and purpose of these undertakings as we begin to examine the progress that has occurred.

## References

Cutler, Neal E., and Robert A. Harootyan. Demography of the Aged. In Woodruff, Diana S., and James E. Birren (eds.). *Aging: Scientific Perspectives and Social Issues.* New York: D. Van Nostrand, 1975.

Drucker, Peter F. *The Unseen Revolution: How Pension Fund Socialism Came to America.* New York: Harper and Row, 1976.

Powell, F.C. *Programs and Services for the Elderly.* New York: Springer, 1979.

Rockstein, Morris, Jeffrey A. Chesky, and Marvin L. Sussman. Comparative Biology and Evolution of Aging. In Finch, Caleb E., and Leonard Hayflick (eds.). *Handbook of the Biology of Aging.* New York: Van Nostrand Reinhold, 1976.

Siegel, Jacob S. *Demographic Aspects of Aging and the Older Population in the United States.* Current Population Reports, Special Studies Series, p. 23 No. 59. Washington, D.C.: Bureau of Census, U.S. Department of Commerce, 1976.

Woodruff, Diana S. Introduction: Multidisciplinary Perspectives of Aging. In Woodruff, Diana S., and James E. Birren (eds.). *Aging: Scientific Perspectives and Social Issues.* New York: D. Van Nostrand, 1975.

# 2

# Growing Awareness of the Aging in Higher Education

Institutions of higher education are not removed from developments of the larger society. As faculty, students, governing boards, and administrators attempt to understand and improve the human condition, they interact with and respond to their milieu. This response may not develop smoothly or consistently, often preceding or trailing societal events. There is a continuing tension of catching up or pulling society along in order to bring into line the perceptions of society and academe. This has been especially true of the area of aging. Some faculty participated in the community and national movements that were taking place, although in large part these occurred with only modest assistance from faculty or students. In the early stages, most of the events did not affect colleges and universities; it has been only in recent years that change has been forced upon our educational institutions.

Educational institutions responded to the growing visibility of older people in several ways. First, surveys and descriptive research projects were undertaken which provided data to support the concept that the aging have social problems. Often these studies included the measurement of income inadequacy, the identification of health difficulties, and the documentation of isolation among this segment of the population. These data were typically used in the political and social policy process in order to show the deplorable substandard conditions under which many older people live. Many studies were generated by a desire to raise the community's awareness of the current level of living and by doing so encourage the development of new social programs and services. Others emanated from a desire to understand the contemporary conditions of the older population and in some ways were simply attempts to expand the knowledge base in sociology, demography, economics, or social psychology.

The second response took the form of research designed to understand the social and psychological processes of later life. Studies were undertaken on retirement adjustment, the effect of the loss of a spouse, and the changes in roles that occur in later life. The measurement of cognitive change became popular, and extensive data were collected in laboratory studies on the ability of persons of different ages to learn specific tasks and content. In most cases, there was a fusion of basic and applied research as educators and practitioners attempted to use the knowledge gained to benefit older people. In much research the application of multidisciplinary approaches was used and has resulted in broader and more insightful results of the projects undertaken.

A review of these developments will provide an understanding of the involvement of institutions of higher education in generating knowledge and applying it to the older population. This involves research development, publication of major works, establishment of scholarly associations, and the founding of several programs in major educational institutions.

## Development of Research in Aging

Although poets, authors, and playwrights have shown awareness of the older population for centuries, physical and social scientists have only recently begun to explore the complex and interactive processes of aging. The earliest studies, undertaken in the late 1800s and the early 1900s, included aging as an incidental variable in experiments on plants and animals. Aging considerations were not the major thrusts of the research, and comparative data on young and old organisms were more a by-product than a purpose of early investigations. This is not surprising, because a life-span developmental perspective had not been conceptualized and an understanding of the organism as static or homeostatic was necessary before the dynamic elements could be introduced.

A few early studies, however, did concentrate on one aspect of aging. Works such as Minot's *The Problems of Age, Growth and Death* (1908), Metchnikoff's *The Prolongation of Life* (1908), Child's *Senescence and Rejuvenescence* (1915), and Pearl's *Biology of Death*

(1922) dealt with the physical and biological aspects of later life. Although each of these works had some drawbacks such as weak theory, inaccuracy, or incompleteness (Birren and Clayton, 1975), they made a major contribution in attracting the attention of researchers to the later stages of life and indicating that a distinction could be made between the pathological disease states that often occur in later life and the normal processes of aging.

Early medical studies also revealed an interest in aging-related events. E. V. Cowdry's book *Arteriosclerosis: A Survey of the Problem*, published in 1933, initiated the examination of relationships between blood circulation and aging, research which presaged today's understanding of the importance of diet in the continued health of people of all ages. This research direction suggested for the first time that the processes of aging might be controlled or modified through planned intervention based on knowledge. Previous assumptions had held that growing old could be controlled only through magic, rituals, or potions (see Segerberg, 1975). Awareness was dawning that at least some of the accompaniments of aging could be reduced, slowed, or eliminated through planned action and preventive health techniques.

G. Stanley Hall is credited with writing one of the first major works on the psychological process of aging. Although he had spent his life studying adolescents, as he approached retirement he became concerned about the later years. His book *Senescence, the Second Half of Life* (1922) indicated that old age was not the inverse of childhood but was a period of life with its own unique aspects—its own feelings, thoughts, and motivations. He concluded that old age was a period of great variability and that individual differences are probably greater than those in youth (Birren and Clayton, 1975). He expanded his studies into the areas of religious behavior and death expectation and reported unique findings in these areas, too. It had been assumed that people became more religious with age because they feared impending death. His studies showed no increase in religious interest or fear of death in old age (Birren, 1961). These findings opened the avenue of cohort analysis, which has shown that differences between young and old people may not be age related but are instead related to the time at which the individual was socialized.

In the late 1920s, Stanford University established the first major research unit devoted to study of the psychological aspects of later life. The Later Maturity Project under the direction of Walter R. Miles was supported by the Josiah Macy Foundation and initiated experimental work with older people in the San Francisco Bay area. The project resulted in a chapter in the 1933 publication *Problems of Aging,* edited by Cowdry. For the first time, psychology took an equal place beside biology, physiology, and medicine as a legitimate area of aging study (Tibbitts, 1960; Geist, 1968).

Another approach to the psychological changes was undertaken by Lehman (1953), who studied productivity over the life span by enumerating the outstanding contributions of scientists and scholars at different ages. By this process, he discovered that persons in several scholarly fields did their best work in the decade between their 30th and 40th birthdays (Kimmel, 1974; Birren, 1964), but that productivity was maintained in some fields well into the sixth and seventh decades of life. Thus, he provided the first empirical data indicating that creativity and productivity did not necessarily decrease in later life but that under certain circumstances could be maintained, cultivated, and expanded.

Between 1920 and 1960, psychologists began to develop a life-span view of personality development. Instead of considering personality to be formed exclusively by inheritance or by the environment of the childhood years, several psychologists began to examine the interactions of genetic predispositions and environmental determinants and developed concepts of a life-long process in which personality continues to change and grow. Persons like Charlotte Buhler, Else Frenkel-Brunswik, Erik Erikson, and Robert Havighurst formulated personality and behavior descriptions that not only differentiated the stages of childhood and adolescence, but delineated the tasks and possibilities that exist in middle age and later life (Kimmel, 1974). These theories provided an awareness of the dynamic nature of later maturity and gave impetus to therapeutic and educational approaches designed to assist older people to adjust, grow, and actualize.

This developmental framework provided the underpinnings for two major longitudinal research efforts. The first was the Kansas City Study of Adult Life, undertaken by the faculty of the Committee on Human Development of the University of Chicago. Using two panels of respondents, 50 to 70 years and 70 to 90 years of age, middle- and working-class people in Kansas City, Missouri, were interviewed seven times over a six-year period to ascertain developmental trends in behavior during the later stages of life (Havighurst, Neugarten, and Tobin, 1968).

This study resulted in one of the most controversial and best-known books of the period, Cummings and Henry's *Growing Old:*

*The Process of Disengagement* (1961). It concluded that there is a natural sociopsychological process in which the individual and society draw apart in the later stages of life. The well-adjusted individual may be expected to disengage, this withdrawal resulting in positive benefits to both the older person and society. This disengagement theory of aging has been attacked, revised, and discussed more than any other position in the history of gerontology. Today, there is little support for it as the definitive explanation for behavior in later life; however, it remains useful in understanding the behavioral contractions common to many older people and apparently the expectation of society generally.

The second longitudinal study examined the changes that typically occur in the later stages of life from a somewhat broader perspective. Faculty of the Center for Aging and Human Development at Duke University began a study in 1954 to investigate the physical, mental, and social processes of aging among normal community residents. A sample of 256 persons over the age of 60 was interviewed and examined on several occasions during a 15-year period. The reports of this research provide baseline data on normal intellectual functioning, family behavior, life satisfaction, attitudes toward aging, medical problems, and mental health problems of older people outside of institutions (Palmore, 1970).

During the 1930s and 1940s, the first sociologically oriented works on aging began to appear. A study published by Landis in 1940 described the "Attitudes and Adjustments of Aged Rural People in Iowa" and began the process of differentiation among the various subgroups of older persons in the population. This differentiation provided understanding of the extensive diversity within the older population, not only among individuals, but among social groups as well. Leo W. Simmons' monumental book, *The Role of the Aged in Primitive Society* (1945), set the stage for the study of the effect on older people of the transition from an agrarian to an industrial society (Tibbitts, 1960). It is now clear that the level of social development of a society has a major effect on the roles and status of older people. Those nations that are highly modernized not only have more older people but treat them quite differently than do developing nations (Cowgill, 1974).

The 1940s also saw the development of the first collective planning for the development of research in the sociology of aging. In 1943 Dr. E. W. Burgess, chairman of the Social Science Research Council's Committee on Social Adjustment, established a Committee on Social Adjustment in Old Age and appointed Robert Havighurst to head it. This committee's work culminated in a 1948 report by Otto Pollack entitled *Social Adjustment in Old Age*. This work not only summarized the state of the art at that time but identified areas of research such as attitudes and adjustment to retirement that have guided much of the sociological research undertaken in the subsequent years (Pollack, 1948).

The more recent emphases in higher education research and publication have focused on the interdisciplinary nature of the field. This direction was initiated when Harold E. Jones edited and published the proceedings of a conference held in Berkeley in 1950. This book clearly interrelated the biological, sociological, demographic, political, and economic aspects of aging (Maddox and Wiley, 1976) and showed for the first time the necessity to reach beyond any single discipline in order to gain an adequate breadth of perspective. This multidisciplinary focus was extended by two major works published in the late 1960s. The first, *Middle Age and Aging* by Bernice Neugarten (1968), provided a comprehensive overview of psychological, sociopsychological, and social research on the middle and later portions of the life span. It brought together the best published articles in a single source, still widely used as a text and reader.

The second, *Aging and Society: Volume I—An Inventory of Research Findings* edited by Riley and Foner (1968), chronicled in a unique but very usable format existing empirical research on many social scientific aspects of aging. This book served as an encyclopedia of the research findings in the field of aging and became a major reference source, still of great value to authors, researchers, and practitioners. These books marked the beginning of attempts to bring the existing knowledge in the field into some organized framework which could be taught in an organized manner. This development had been initiated by the original Handbooks on Aging, to be discussed in a later section, which for the first time provided the multidisciplinary interrelationships necessary for understanding the broad parameters of the field.

In 1976–77 the compilation of knowledge in the field was updated through the publication of three new handbooks: *Handbook of Aging and the Social Sciences* (Binstock & Shanas), *Handbook of the Biology of Aging* (Finch & Hayflick), and *Handbook of the Psychology of Aging* (Birren & Schaie). These provide the most up-to-date, comprehensive review of research and theory in the field and show the great expansion in the quantity and quality of research accomplished during the 17 years between the first and second sets of handbooks. No researcher, however, would assert that enough is now known; much is still unclear or totally obscure, and extensive research remains to be conducted in the separate areas of inquiry, as well as in the application of this knowledge to the current needs of older people in this nation and around the world.

Research and publication in the area of aging, then, have experienced significant growth during this century. From almost no work having been done before 1900, we can now find literally thousands of citations in a variety of fields related to both the traditional disciplines and the professions. Riegel (1973) reported that the number of publications on aging averaged only four or five per year in 1920, while the number reached nearly 250 annually by 1970. Birren and Clayton (1975) report that between 1900 and 1949 a total of five or six books per year were published which dealt with aging. They found that between 1950 and 1960 as much literature on aging was produced as was published during the preceding 100 years, and they predicted that the amount would at least double during the decade of the 1970s.

Thus, it becomes obvious that researchers and writers, primarily from institutions of higher education, have become much more aware of the growth and importance of the phenomenon of aging and have increasingly focused interest and research on the processes of aging and the condition of contemporary older people.

## Establishment of Professional Organizations

Just as the publication of major books in the area indicated the development of a body of knowledge that could be compiled and shared, the development of scholarly and professional organizations indicated that researchers in the field were beginning to identify their interests in aging as important and worthy of sharing with others who had similar motivations.

Perhaps the first scholarly organization specifically in the area was the International Club for Research on Aging, established by British scientists in 1939. In that same year, the American Research Club was organized with the support of the Josiah Macy Foundation. This group met for several years and in 1945 incorporated as the Gerontological Society, an organization designed to promote scientific study of aging and to unite the activities of gerontologists working in various scientific fields as well as those responsible for the care and treatment of the aged (Adler, 1958). Its publications, the *Journal of Gerontology* (begun in 1946) and the *Gerontologist* (1960), provide the major mechanisms for researchers and policy makers to share their findings and conceptualizations on the current state of the field.

The Gerontological Society remains the major professional/scientific organization on aging. Its membership, now over 4,200, represents academics as well as program planners, policy makers, clinicians, and community practitioners. Although maintaining a strong interest in the physiological and medical aspects of the field, it is clear that the membership is now heavily dominated by persons who are more concerned with program and policy. This has occurred because the number of jobs in community programs has rapidly outpaced positions in institutions of higher education, research centers, and clinics.

Researchers and practitioners from a number of nations showed their interest in common problems by establishing the International Association of Gerontology in 1950 in Liège, Belgium. That organization has conducted conferences every third year to encourage international exchange of ideas and facilitate increased closeness among professionals of many nations. The organization remains vital and attendance at its meetings continues to grow.

The American Psychological Association was one of the first national scientific organizations to recognize aging as a major area of concern for many of its members. In 1946 that organization created the Division on Maturity and Old Age, which facilitated interest in the area by conducting a survey of course work in gerontology in 1948. It also sponsored a major conference, which resulted in the publication of John Anderson's book, *Psychological Aspects of Aging* (Donahue, 1967). Although early membership in the Division was limited, recent years have seen a great growth, and it is clear that psychologists now recognize research and training in aging as an important part of the field (Schaie, 1978).

Regional organizations in gerontology are also becoming increasingly visible. The oldest, the Western Gerontological Society, was established nearly 25 years ago and now numbers over 2,500 members. It is a strong source of information sharing and mutual support for practitioners, older people, and educators in the western third of the nation. Its publications and annual meetings appeal to the program- and policy-oriented person, and as the public programs for aging have grown, so has the size and vitality of the organization. Regional organizations are now in the formative stages in other parts of the country.

A major interuniversity program in the sociological area was initiated in 1961 when the Midwest Council for Social Research on Aging was formed. This organization, composed originally of nine member universities from the Great Plains region, has encouraged pre- and postdoctoral training in aging at the member schools and remains active in stimulating research and advanced training in relation to aging (Donahue, 1967).

The most recently formed of the organizations in the field is the Association for Gerontology in Higher Education, which offers membership to colleges and universities with programs in aging. Begun as an ad hoc committee in 1972, the organization was incorporated in 1974 and now has a membership of more than 150 institutions that have banded together to develop and improve gerontology education (Hickey, 1978). This group is currently undertaking the development of data collection that may lead to the setting of some general expectations for instruction in gerontology. Other major activities have been the conducting of several conferences on gerontology education, the publication of a book of conference papers entitled *Gerontology in Higher Education: Perspectives and Issues* (Seltzer, et al., 1978), and the provision of assistance to many colleges and universities that desire to begin instructional programs in this area.

## Inter-University Training Program

One of the major events in the development of the field was the establishment of the Inter-University Training Program in Gerontology. In 1955 the Psychological and Social Sciences Section of the Gerontological Society formed a committee to explore roles of the social sciences in studying aging. The committee was composed of three of the major figures in the development of gerontology—James Birren, Wilma Donahue, and Clark Tibbitts. Their committee reported back to the section that additional training in gerontology was needed within the institutions of higher education in this country and that to achieve this end, it would be necessary to conduct in-service education of faculty members so that they could gain the necessary orientation to the field.

A committee composed of Robert Kleemeier, Ewald Busse, John Anderson, and Ernest Burgess was established to implement Birren, Donahue, and Tibbitts' recommendations. A conference to begin the planning and development process was held at the University of Michigan in 1956. This meeting ended in the agreement that an interuniversity project would be undertaken and that it would be administratively housed at the University of Michigan with Wilma Donahue as project director.

With financial support from the National Institute of Mental Health and the National Heart Institute, four major activities were decided upon. The first involved a survey of current instruction in the field of aging at institutions of higher education. Of 312 colleges and universities responding to a mailed questionnaire, only 50 offered credit courses in any aspect of gerontology and only 72 could identify any research underway. The conclusion was drawn that additional research and instruction were needed; the other three activities of the interuniversity program were designed to support and encourage this development.

The second activity involved the compilation of current knowledge in the area of gerontology. This took the form of three major handbooks which were, at that time, the most complete and authoritative sources available. The first to be completed (1959) was edited by James Birren and was entitled the *Handbook of Aging and the Individual: Psychological and Biological Aspects of Aging.* The second (1960), the *Handbook of Social Gerontology: Societal Aspects of Aging,* was edited by Clark Tibbitts and not only dealt with the social aspects of aging but laid down the basic concepts of the field of social gerontology for the first time. The third book, *Aging in Western Societies: A Survey of Social Gerontology* (1960), was edited by Ernest Burgess and provided a comparison of the aging-related aspects of several cultures.

The third activity of the project was the development of curriculum guides in five areas: psychology of aging, sociology of aging, social welfare and the aged, economics of an aging population, and an interdisciplinary course in social gerontology. These syllabi were developed by highly respected persons and were widely distributed to college and university faculty desiring to initiate course work. They not only became the basis of many courses developed during the early 1960s, but they also served as models of what course work in gerontology should be during these developmental years.

The fourth activity was to conduct two summer workshops for faculty who would be involved in gerontology education. It was concluded that the way to fill the immediate need for faculty to teach and conduct research in aging was to involve current faculty in the area in workshops that provided an introduction to the content and an exposure to existing resources, needs, and personnel. The workshops were held at the University of California at Berkeley in 1958 and University of Connecticut in 1959. The 36 to 40 participants selected were from colleges and universities across the country; many of these persons did indeed become the initiators of activities at their institutions of higher education.

The interuniversity training program, then, was a major impetus to the development of gerontology education in colleges and universities. The materials, syllabi, and faculty training began to change the focus from research on specific aspects of the field to the preparation of researchers and teachers, as well as of practitioners who would provide services to older people. The results have been long lasting. The Handbooks were the primary source of content for many years, and the syllabi were used until faculty began to feel secure in modifying courses to fit their own special interests. The majority of fellows in the summer institutes did offer courses and/or directed research in gerontology (Donahue, 1960).

## Institutional Program Development

The development of research and education programs in colleges has been heavily dependent upon two factors: the interest and leadership of a key faculty member or administrator and the availability of financial support from outside the institution.

The emergence of gerontology as a subject of study at the college level occurred at a time (1967 to the present) when many institutions were unable to allocate internal resources for program expansion. The only way that expansion could occur was through the use of funds from other sources. The federal government thus became the principal provider of funds and therefore set the direction for gerontology programs. As resources became available, more and more colleges showed an interest in the field and developed programs more comprehensive than the mere conducting of a research project or offering of a class. It is possible to describe this development in four sequential stages that closely parallel changes in the availability of funds from several federal agencies.

The first stage of gerontology education occurred before 1966 and involved the founding of viable programs of training in research at a few major institutions, supported by funds from the National Institute of Mental Health and the National Institute of Child Health and Human Development. The main thrust was for doctoral level training for students interested in research and teaching careers in the field of aging. The funding provided faculty support and stipends for only a small number of students at a very few universities, but it did begin the process of building a cadre of personnel which could be expanded as subsequent funding became available.

The second stage was initiated when the U.S. Administration on Aging (HEW) began its career training grant program during 1966 and 1967. Funds were made available under the Older Americans Act to prepare practitioners for jobs to be created by community programs sponsored by the Act. Several colleges and universities received funding for faculty and student support; instruction at the master's degree level was initiated in many human service professions: social work, public administration, education, health, and housing management. Some of this support went to universities with previous NIH support, while some went to institutions establishing gerontology activities for the first time.

In 1972–73 the third expansion occurred when AoA reopened competitive career training grants. From 1967 to 1972, Congressional appropriations had remained fixed so existing projects were re-funded annually, but few new ones were approved. In 1972 expansion of funding occurred and several more universities and colleges received support. For the first time several undergraduate  programs were initiated and instruction at predominantly black or minority colleges was funded. This expansion allowed for the development of training programs in most states and resulted in a substantial increase in the number and diversity of graduates.

Finally, in 1976–77, Title IV-C of the Older Americans Act, providing for multidisciplinary centers of aging, was funded and allowed a further expansion of activities and programs. This title encouraged the planning and implementation of multifaceted programs of research, service, and education to be developed at several universities. A number of these grants went to the universities and colleges which had already had other grants for some years, but others were awarded to higher education institutions which had theretofore not been deeply involved in gerontology. Thus, thanks to government interest and funding, the breadth and quality of instruction programs has been substantially increased.

This financial support from the Administration on Aging was preceded by research and training grants from the National Institute on Child Health and Human Development. In 1974 these programs were transferred to the newly established National Institute on Aging, whose major purpose is to conduct and support biomedical, social, and behavioral research related to the aging processes and diseases as well as to other special problems and needs of the aged. Current support for extramural research and training-for-research projects is aimed at the causes and mechanisms of aging, medical problems of aging, and psychosocial problems of the elderly.

The early stages of gerontology development in institutions of higher education followed a fairly discernible pattern. First, one or two faculty members or students conducted research that raised additional questions about the processes of aging and older people. This research aroused interest in other students or faculty members, in turn creating the need for more resources, which in its turn opened further opportunities for research, and so on and on, in a widening spiral, eventually resulting in the establishment of some administrative or academic unit which focused its major energy on the topic of aging. This unit could then provide the necessary visibility to attract quality students and additional funding. Four early entrants into the field of gerontology can be identified as having followed this pattern: the University of Chicago, the University of Michigan, Duke University, and the University of Southern California.

The University of Chicago was one of the first institutions of higher education to become involved. Ernest Burgess and Robert Havighurst have already been identified as key figures in the Social Science Research Council's pioneering activities. Within their own institution, they developed several research projects and encouraged student interest in the later stages of life. This activity led to the formation of the Committee on Human Development in 1957, which continues to provide an academic home for students and faculty interested in fundamental research on aging. Burgess, Havighurst, Bernice Neugarten, and Sheldon Tobin developed the program, which remains an outstanding example of interdisciplinary commitment to research in aging (Donahue, 1967).

The University of Michigan began conducting studies on the needs of older people in 1948, under the direction of Clark Tibbitts. A series of annual conferences, initiated the same year, took on a national stature by bringing together researchers and policy makers to examine specific problem areas in services to and conditions of older people. The proceedings of several of the conferences were published, providing a continuing supply of up-to-date information for the new educational programs that were developing at that time. Wilma Donahue, who became chairman of Michigan's Division of Gerontology of the Institute for Human Adjustment in 1950, directed that program and the Institute of Gerontology (established in 1965) for nearly 20 years, until her retirement.

Duke University was also an early leader in developing gerontology research. In 1954 Ewald Busse initiated a series of studies on the relationship of physiological, psychological, and social factors in aging. The involvement of several faculty members in these studies led to the establishment of the Regional Center for the Study of Aging (1957), which later became the Center for the Study of Aging and Human Development. The Center enjoys a history of high-quality medical-psychological research, which has been expanded to include longitudinal studies on the normal processes of aging (Donahue, 1967). Carl Eisdorfer and George Maddox subsequently directed the program, which has attained international stature.

Finally, the University of Southern California was an early entrant in the area of gerontology education with the establishment of the Roosmoor-Cortese Institute for the Study of Retirement and Aging (1964). James Birren, the Institute's first director, developed a center, renamed the Ethel Percy Andrus Gerontology Center in honor of the founder and first president of the American Association of Retired Persons/National Retired Teacher's Association. The center, housed in a new and well-equipped laboratory/office building, is today one of the largest gerontology research, service, and education centers in the world. Dr. Birren continues as director and as dean of the Leonard Davis School of Gerontology, founded in 1975.

The availability of career training grants from the Administration on Aging provided the major impetus for expansion of gerontology education programs in the past 10 years. These funds were used for the creation and operation of "training" programs to prepare future professionals for planning, implementation, and administration of community services for older people. Although most of the 1966 and 1967 grants were awarded to existing programs in social work, public administration, or education, the University of South Florida (at Tampa) and North Texas State University (at Denton) used the funds to develop master's degree programs in gerontology which emphasized social service and housing administration, respectively. Universities such as Wayne State, Arizona, Minnesota, Brandeis, Columbia, North Carolina, Oregon, and Wisconsin received career training grants at this time and developed substantial programs, most of which continue to offer professional preparation for graduate students.

In 1972 an additional group of institutions was awarded career grants as the funding was expanded. Most of these institutions had little previous background in the field but committed activity in gerontology has resulted. This group of programs engendered more diversity of discipline and profession and brought gerontology into numerous departments. Universities such as UCLA, Miami (of Ohio), Maryland, Boston, Nebraska, SUNY, Case Western Reserve, Oregon State, Portland State, Pennsylvania, Pittsburgh, Pennsylvania State, Fisk, and Washington were added to the growing list with organized programs in the field.

The 1976–77 expansion of funding added another group of colleges and universities, many of which had a long research record but less involvement in the preparation of professionals for service delivery. Institutions such as Florida State, Illinois (Chicago Circle), Iowa, Hawaii, Connecticut, Alabama, Miami, Kentucky, Louisville, Temple, San Diego State, Akron, Hampton, Wichita State, Virginia Commonwealth, Puerto Rico, Kansas, West Virginia, and Missouri received support. These universities, as well as others that have over the years received research, technical assistance, or continuing education funding, represent the substantial increase in participating institutions. There remain, however, hundreds of universities with little or no activity in aging, and most smaller four-year and community colleges have no courses at all.         *small = less ger*

## Conclusions

The demographic and social trends that increased the visibility of older persons in the United States has encouraged the federal government to create social, health, and income maintenance programs designed to alleviate problems and improve the quality of life for older citizens. These programs have substantially increased the number and level of jobs in human services for older people and have clearly shown the need for greater quality of information on the basic elements of aging.

Institutions of higher education have responded to these events by conducting research on the basic and applied nature of aging and by developing curricula to prepare individuals for administrative, service, and research roles in government and private agencies. These instructional programs have led to the establishment of several gerontology centers, institutes, programs, or departments now institutionalized in many colleges and universities. Government funding is directing this development toward professional and applied concerns, and it may be expected that the future will hold more in the way of practice-oriented research and instruction.

# References

Adler, Marjorie. History of Gerontological Society, Inc. *Journal of Gerontology*, 1958, *13*, 94–102.

Anderson, J. E. (ed.). *Psychological Aspects of Aging*. Washington, D.C.: American Psychological Association, 1956.

Binstock, R. H. and E. Shanas (eds.). *Handbook of Aging and the Social Sciences*. New York: Van Nostrand Reinhold, 1976.

Birren, James E. A Brief History of the Psychology of Aging. *The Gerontologist*, 1961, *1*, 67–77.

Birren, James E. (ed.). *Handbook of Aging and the Individual*. Chicago: University of Chicago Press, 1959.

Birren, James E. *The Psychology of Aging*. Englewood Cliffs, N.J.: Prentice-Hall, 1964.

Birren, James E., and Vivian Clayton. History of Gerontology. In Woodruff, Diane S., and James E. Birren (eds.). *Aging: Scientific Perspectives and Social Issues*. New York: D. Van Nostrand, 1975.

Birren, James E. and K. W. Schaie (eds.). *Handbook of the Psychology of Aging*. New York: Van Nostrand Reinhold, 1977.

Burgess, Ernest W. (ed.). *Aging in Western Societies: A Survey of Social Gerontology*. Chicago: University of Chicago Press, 1960.

Child, C. M. *Senescence and Rejuvenescence*. Chicago: University of Chicago Press, 1915.

Cowdry, E. V. (ed.). *Arteriosclerosis: A Survey of the Problem*. Josiah Macy, Jr. Foundation N.Y. New York: MacMillan, 1933.

Cowdry, E. V. (ed.). *Problems of Aging*. Baltimore: Walhams and Wilkins, 1939.

Cowgill, Donald O. The Aging of Populations and Societies. *The Annals of the American Academy of Political and Social Science: Political Consequences of Aging*, 1974, *415*, 1–18.

Cummings, E. M. and W. E. Henry. *Growing Old: The Process of Disengagement*. New York: Basic Books, 1961.

Donahue, Wilma. Development and Current Status of University Instruction in Social Gerontology. In Kushner, Rose E., and Marion E. Bunch (eds.). *Graduate Education in Aging within the Social Sciences*. Ann Arbor, Mich.: University of Michigan Division of Gerontology, 1967.

Donahue, Wilma. Training in Social Gerontology. *Geriatrics*, 1960, *15*, 801–809.

Finch, C. E. and L. Hayflick (eds.). *Handbook of the Biology of Aging*. New York: Van Nostrand Reinhold, 1977.

Geist, Harold. *The Psychological Aspects of the Aging Process: With Sociological Implications*. St. Louis: Warren H. Green, 1968.

Hall, G. S. *Senescence, the Second Half of Life*. New York: Appleton, 1922.

Havighurst, Robert J., Bernice L. Neugarten, and Sheldon S. Tobin. Disengagement and Patterns of Aging. In Bernice L. Neugarten (ed.). *Middle Age and Aging.* Chicago: University of Chicago Press, 1968.

Hickey, Tom. Association for Gerontology in Higher Education—A Brief History. In Mildred M. Seltzer, Harvey Sterns, and Tom Hickey (eds.). *Gerontology in Higher Education: Perspectives and Issues.* Belmont, Calif.: Wadsworth Publishing, 1978.

Kimmel, Douglas C. *Adulthood and Aging.* New York: John Wiley and Sons, 1974.

Landis, J. T. Attitudes and Adjustments of Aged Rural People in Iowa. Unpublished Ph.D. dissertation, Louisiana State University, 1940.

Lehman, H. C. *Age and Achievement.* Princeton, N. J.: Princeton University Press, 1953.

Maddox, George L., and James Wiley. Scope, Concepts, and Methods in the Study of Aging. In Binstock, Robert H., and Ethel Shanas (eds.). *Handbook of Aging and the Social Sciences.* New York: Van Nostrand Reinhold, 1976.

Metchnikoff, E. *The Prolongation of Life.* New York: Putnam and Sons, 1908.

Minot, C. *The Problems of Age, Growth, and Death.* New York: Putnam and Sons, 1908.

Neugarten, B. L. (ed.). *Middle Age and Aging.* Chicago: The University of Chicago Press, 1968.

Palmore Erdman (ed.). *Normal Aging.* Durham, N.C.: Duke University Press, 1970.

Pearl, R. *The Biology of Death.* Philadelphia: J.P. Lippincott, 1922.

Pollack, Otto. *Social Adjustment in Old Age: A Research Planning Report.* New York: Social Science Research Council, 1948.

Riegel, Klaus F. On the History of Psychological Gerontology. In Eisdorfer, Carl and M. Powell Lawton (eds.). *The Psychology of Adult Development and Aging.* Washington, D.C.: American Psychological Association, 1973.

Riley, M. W. and Anne Foner. *Aging and Society: Volume One—An Inventory of Research Findings.* New York: Russell Sage Foundation, 1968.

Schaie, K. Warner. Great Issues in Academic Gerontology: Where Are We Going and Why? In Mildred M. Seltzer, Harvey Sterns, and Tom Hickey (eds.). *Gerontology in Higher Education: Perspectives and Issues.* Belmont, Calif.: Wadsworth Publishing, 1978.

Segerberg, Osborn, Jr. *The Immortality Factor.* New York: Bantam Books, 1975.

Seltzer, Mildred M., Harvey Sterns, and Tom Hickey (eds.). *Gerontology in Higher Education: Perspectives and Issues.* Belmont, Calif.: Wadsworth Publishing, 1978.

Simmons, L. W. *The Role of the Aged in Primitive Society.* New Haven, Conn.: Yale University Press, 1945.

Tibbitts, Clark (ed.). *Handbook of Social Gerontology: Societal Aspects of Aging*. Chicago: University of Chicago Press, 1960. ) Key

Tibbitts, Clark. Origin, Scope, and Fields of Social Gerontology. In Clark Tibbitts (ed.). *Handbook of Social Gerontology: Societal Aspects of Aging*. Chicago: University of Chicago Press, 1960.

# 3

# The Literature of
# Gerontology Education

Gerontology education has developed rapidly during the past 15 years. Course work, programs of instruction, and institutional arrangements have been established with the purpose of facilitating the dissemination of knowledge about the processes of aging and assisting students to acquire professional skills useful in planning and providing services to older people. These developments have occurred within a short period of time and in a variety of institutions; there is currently limited consistency in the organizational structures, curricula, staffing, and program outcomes. Even the terminology used varies from one institution to another, causing confusion in attempts to assess the current state of development.

In order to avoid misunderstanding, it is appropriate at this juncture to define three terms which will be often used and which are likely to have varying meanings. These are *social gerontology, educational gerontology,* and *gerontology education*.

The term *social gerontology,* widely recognized today within the field of aging, is generally considered to be concerned with the interaction between the behavioral aspects of aging and aging as a social phenomenon. Tibbitt's *Handbook of Social Gerontology* (1960) defined the parameters of this field of study and suggested that social gerontology might evolve into a discipline with content drawn from the social, behavioral, and political sciences. Social gerontology concentrates on the social and psychological attributes of aging but does not exclude the biological and physiological aspects.

The term *educational gerontology* is newer and less familiar to persons in gerontology. It denotes the study and practice of educa-

28

tional approaches to improving the quality of life for older people. Typically it includes such areas as the education of older people, education of the public about older people, and education of professionals and practitioners who will work with older people (Peterson, 1976). Education of older people has expanded extensively as adult and continuing education programs have recognized retirees as a potential audience and have initiated lecture and discussion programs on their behalf. As a part of the area of lifelong learning, education for and about older people can be expected to remain a growth field in the future.

This chapter deals with one of the aspects of educational gerontology—*gerontology education*. This term denotes the credit instruction of students at the undergraduate and graduate levels on the condition of the older population and the processes of aging. For some students this instruction will comprise preparation for a job (professional or vocational education), for others it will offer an understanding of one aspect of the contemporary world (academic education), while for some it will involve preparation for research and teaching (scientific education).

It will be noted that the continuing education of professionals and practitioners who are currently employed in planning, administration, or service positions in agencies serving older people is not included within this definition of gerontology education, although it would certainly be possible to do so. There is much activity in this area well worth evaluation and review, but it is peripheral to the primary intent of this work.

A substantial amount of gerontology education literature has been produced in the past few years, scattered throughout numerous periodicals and books and somewhat uneven in quality and specificity. A survey of this literature will provide an understanding of the major concepts as well as indicate the distribution across the possible interest areas.

With even a limited review four major categories of emphasis become apparent: (1) gerontology as a discipline, including the rationale for and activities directed toward the creation of a separate body of knowledge and service delivery system for gerontology; (2) the need for gerontology content to be included in other fields of instruction, especially professional fields; (3) gerontology content and outcomes as a part of the academic education offered in undergraduate and graduate programs; and (4) the development of a profession of gerontology and the need for trained manpower to provide services to older people.

These four topics include most of the current writing in gerontology education. Since the field is yet in its infancy, there is limited
consensus in numerous areas and the reader should not be concerned
if conflicts appear in this review. These conflicts exist in reality and
may well be beneficial. Seltzer (1974) has observed that the diversity
of the field sometimes verges on chaos, but since this is a period of
growth and formulation, rapid solidification of structures, curricula,
and outcomes would be premature and unwise. Some of the less
successful and less efficient approaches may well "shake out" in time,
resulting in a better program than would be possible if disagreement
were discouraged prematurely.

## Gerontology as a Discipline

Gerontology is a multidisciplinary field; content and methods are
drawn from biology, medical science, psychology, sociology, economics, political science, education, and the social services. Whether
this content is best transmitted through an integrated sequence of
courses offered within a gerontology department or whether individual courses should be conducted within several departments so that
aging is examined from the point of view of a particular discipline or
profession remains, however, an open question.

One early approach to the situation was an attempt to establish
gerontology as an "interdisciplinary discipline." This method, which
went through two distinct stages, continues to be a viable approach
to organizing gerontology instruction. In the 1960s Wilma Donahue
and Clark Tibbitts became advocates for this approach, encouraging
several actions that led toward the development of an independent
field (Tibbitts, 1960), including the Inter-University Training Program in Social Gerontology, an attempt to define the field, outline
the curricula, prepare materials, and train instructors (Donahue,
1960).

Support for a discipline of gerontology was articulated by Robert
Kleemeier in his presidential address to the Gerontological Society,
in which he emphasized the need for a unique field of gerontology
that would be buttressed by the growing visibility of older people in
this nation and an increasing awareness of their needs and problems.
He suggested that if aging were viewed as a destructive process, then
the needs of older people would require the assistance of a discipline
devoted to studying and ameliorating the effects of aging. He also
emphasized the shortage of trained manpower to carry out govern-

ment programs such as Medicare, Medicaid, and Social Security. Finally, he indicated the importance of research directed at the needs and conditions of the elderly rather than viewing age as only one of many variables to be considered in research (Kleemeier, 1965). It is apparent in Kleemeier's comments that the discipline was not to be exclusively devoted to seeking truth about the processes of aging but was also to involve meeting the needs of older people through social programs and the preparation of manpower to staff these programs. Thus, although the word *discipline* was consistently used by Donahue, Tibbitts, and Kleemeier, it was defined in a broader and more applied sense than is used in this work.

Tibbitts (1967) moved toward operationalizing the discipline of gerontology by describing the establishment of a service area that would be staffed by a new type of professional called an *applied social gerontologist*. This person would be a gerontological generalist able to communicate and work with professionals in all fields related to aging. He designed a master's degree curriculum in gerontology and outlined the content of several new courses that would be offered.

One step toward implementing this plan occurred when the U.S. Administration on Aging awarded sizable training grants to the University of South Florida and North Texas State University in 1967 for the nation's first master's degree programs in gerontology. In each case the curriculum focused heavily on applied and professional outcomes, with North Texas stressing management of nursing homes and homes for the aged and South Florida emphasizing the planning and delivery of social services. These universities became the proving ground for the planning and conceptualization that had been done in regard to preparation of students for professional service to older people.

Instructional materials for courses in the "discipline" of gerontology were provided by Marvin R. Koller, who edited a book entitled *Social Gerontology* (1968), aimed at the upper-level undergraduate or beginning graduate student. This text not only surveyed the areas of social gerontology in a manner substantially more concise and applied than the earlier handbooks but also described the history and purposes of social gerontology, familiarizing both faculty members and students with the field.

This "disciplinary" approach, however, found only minimal support in most institutions of higher education. Few colleges or universities established actual departments of gerontology or designed the degree programs necessary for the development of professional education. Even the University of Michigan, Wilma Donahue's home institution, decided against creating a degree or department of gerontology. It is only since 1975 that real movement in this direction has occurred, and this typically has resulted not from the belief in the discipline or profession of gerontology, but from other pressures.

One of the major variables in the development of "disciplinary" gerontology education has been the availability of career training grants from the U.S. Administration on Aging. In 1972 Congressional appropriation for this purpose was expanded sufficiently to allow for support of new university and college career training grants; the Administration on Aging encouraged the design of professionally oriented programs that would supply trained manpower for federally funded services for older persons. During the next several years, increasing numbers of institutions chose to better their chances for funding by creating a degree program rather than a specialization in an established department, and consequently, many new degree programs were spawned.

Another motivator toward the establishment of gerontology degrees has been the need for continuing support from the host institution. Since federal money is unlikely to be available indefinitely, most administrators of gerontology education programs began to solicit support from their institutions. Limited resources made this difficult for the college or university unless the gerontology unit could show the permanence and stability of a degree program with its requisite students and credit-hour production. The decentralized approach of spreading gerontology instruction throughout the various departments of the institution did not meet this criterion, so many administrators began the process of gaining support and legitimization for a degree program.

Another aspect of this movement is exemplified by the Leonard Davis School of Gerontology at the University of Southern California, created in 1975. As the first school of gerontology in the nation, its establishment within a widely known and respected gerontology center has attracted national interest. The undergraduate and master's degree programs of the School have come to serve as models for many other institutions. The movement toward a "discipline" has been refocused somewhat toward the creation of degree programs and independent gerontology departments, but the concept remains consistent—that gerontology is best organized and taught as a separate and unique entity.

## Gerontology as an Adjunct Field

Other writers in the area of gerontology education, generally perceived to be the majority, have preferred to see gerontology education as a multidisciplinary supplementation to in-depth instruction within one of the existing disciplines or professions. They would generally prefer to have gerontology course work viewed as an adjunct to instruction in social work, psychology, urban planning, biology, medicine, sociology, education, recreation, or architecture. Thus, the student would receive a degree in the professional or disciplinary field but have some supplementary gerontology course work that would allow him to understand more completely the implications of aging for his chosen field of study (Atchley and Seltzer, n.d.).

Beattie (1974) has been a strong supporter of this position, suggesting that it is not appropriate to train gerontologists per se, but rather to encourage in-depth study within one discipline to be supplemented by knowledge and skill related to the process of aging. He has stressed the importance of administrative and organizational structures that would facilitate this multidisciplinary relationship; the major Center on Aging, which he directs at Syracuse University, is consistent with this philosophical position.

Other authors have identified the value of gerontology education for persons entering professional fields. Social workers, for instance, could use gerontological knowledge to help older persons adapt to those unique and traumatic changes that may occur in later life—retirement, widowhood, relocation, dependency (Johnston, 1974). This knowledge, however, is recommended only for those social workers who have already attained a firm understanding of interpersonal interventions, group processes, and social service delivery systems. The gerontology knowledge is applied in field experiences that bring students into ongoing relationships with older persons in community or institutional settings, typically involving conversations about the philosophical principles raised by older people as they contemplate the meaning of their lives (Lowy and Miller, 1974; Cohen, 1971).

The nursing literature provides a similar view of the value of gerontology education. Although recognition of the need for a specialty in geriatric or gerontic nursing is becoming widely accepted, only recently have comprehensive attempts to define and quantify gerontological nursing instruction been undertaken (Gunter and

Estes, 1978). Curricular design at the baccalaureate and graduate levels indicates the need to understand the physical and social changes that occur in old age which have a relationship to the delivery and reception of health services (McCall, 1974). This type of learning is often encouraged in clinical settings in which nursing students are brought into continued contact with a few older people in order to develop a case history of the older patient (Safier, 1975).

Moberg (1975) has suggested that persons preparing for the clergy are also in need of some special knowledge about older people and the processes of aging. Because nearly half of a typical clergyman's work relates to older people or their families, it is important that the minister be sensitized to the unique needs and problems older people face. Thus, the skills in counseling, visitation, referral, and organization need to be considered in light of the older parishioner. Since few schools of theology currently offer any specific instruction in the area of aging, development of didactic and clinical programs would be most appropriate.

In the area of medical education, several writers have made a similar case. Although geriatric medicine is not a recognized specialty, it is useful for physicians to be exposed to the social and psychological changes of later life and to be sensitized to the special needs of this patient group. This exposure may result in physicians having improved attitudes about older people and providing more empathic services (Chebotarev, 1976; Cohen, 1974; Freeman, 1971; Goldman, 1974; Harris, 1975; Rodstein, 1973).

Gerontological preparation in law schools is also recognized in the literature. The recommended approach is for students to be prepared first in the skills of the law profession and later to be exposed to experiences in which the typical problems of older people are highlighted (Harbaugh, 1976). As in other professions there is little indication that this training is taking place in most American law schools.

Writers from the field of psychology also view gerontology as an adjunct to their discipline. Nevertheless, gerontology instruction in doctoral and postdoctoral psychology programs needs to be expanded to many more universities because graduates will increasingly have the opportunity to provide service to or undertake research with the older population. The emphasis should be placed on the need to provide manpower to work with this clientele group (Birren and Woodruff, 1973) as well as on the need for clinicians and researchers to become more aware of the potential for research and practice in this area (Elias, 1972).

A similar change in attitude is needed in undergraduate study in psychology. Gerontology is viewed at present merely as a special interest area within psychology that may lead to additional employment opportunities or background for advanced study of aging (Hulicka and Morganti, 1976). Community practice or field work experience is typically stressed as especially valuable to undergraduates in gaining exposure to current programs and developing relationships with individual older people.

At this time, instruction provided in connection with degree programs within a profession or discipline is the most common and most widely accepted organizational form of gerontology education. This arrangement assumes that gerontology is not a discipline or profession but rather a specialty area that may be approached through one of the established areas of study. It is inappropriate, according to this view, to offer a degree in gerontology; a preferred alternative is to confer a minor, certificate, or concentration on the student. Literature supporting this position cites several arguments against the development of a degree. These may be summarized as follows:

1. Broad exposure to several disciplinary areas is preferable to a narrow degree focus.

2. Employment opportunities are limited by a degree that prepares the student only for the field of aging.

3. Degree programs compete for scarce university and college resources.

4. There is no current process of accrediting gerontology education programs, so the degree cannot have its quality certified.

5. Gerontology has traditionally meant an eclectic approach and a degree is inconsistent with this position.

6. A degree does not allow for interdisciplinary expansion and broadening of the course work into other disciplines and professions (Baumhover, 1978).

## Gerontology as Academic Instruction

Gerontology instruction originated within the traditional academic disciplines of higher education. Biologists, psychologists, and sociologists were the first to display interest in aging phenomena and develop units of instruction and eventually whole courses around the topic of aging. Since faculty preparation and interest emanated from an academic point of view, it was predictable that early instruction would be oriented toward an empirical description of the processes of aging and the condition of the older population.

This early orientation, maintained in much current instruction, is referred to as *academic gerontology*. It is designed to provide a liberal understanding of the dynamics of the life span developmental processes and an appreciation for these effects on both the individual and society as a whole. Academic gerontology education is described as having four major purposes or emphases: (1) providing content or specific information on the processes of aging or the state of the older person; (2) encouraging students to realize that they too are aging and to consider their own lifelong developmental potential; (3) developing an understanding of the affective elements of aging and the societal attitudes toward older people; and (4) developing intellectual skills of thinking, writing, and research.

In describing the responsibility of the university (and by extension, all of higher education) to the area of gerontology, Ehrlich and Ehrlich (1976) stated that the appropriate purpose of gerontology instruction is to assist students to understand the developments that occur across the life cycle and grasp the meaning these events have for the individual and society. In other words, the desired outcome of gerontology education is a basic understanding of the multifaceted process of aging, of the distinctions between normal and pathological aging, and of the dynamic nature of both individual and cultural aging (Peterson, 1978b). This outlook spares the student, especially the undergraduate, from misplacing energies by imitating professional and graduate programs and integrates gerontology into the traditional liberal goals of higher education (Cooney, 1978).

This liberal arts position is supported by some curricular materials developed recently and widely disseminated such as *An Instructor's Handbook for the Development of a Basic Course in Gerontology* (1975). This monograph outlines an undergraduate course and gives the course objectives as assisting the student to understand aging as it affects the physical, psychological, and social processes of life—a liberal understanding of the developmental aspects of aging.

There is, however, a personal as well as a cognitive side to academic gerontology. Knowledge of the aging process is useful in assisting students to anticipate and adjust appropriately to their own aging. This theme of helping oneself as well as others is widely recognized and is viewed as a supplemental outcome of most gerontology education (Seltzer, 1974). Evaluation of gerontology course work has indicated that constructive, positive knowledge about older people leads to similar attitudes that may facilitate adjustment to the aging process (Hudis, 1974). Thus, knowledge and personal adjustment are two of the clearly desired outcomes of academic gerontology instruction.

A related purpose of academic gerontology concerns the affective realm. It is assumed (and there is much support for the assumption) that many individuals in this society hold negative stereotype beliefs about older people and the processes of aging. These attitudes and beliefs are detrimental to the field of aging because they discourage individuals from supporting programs for the elderly, militate against professional interest in older people as a potential client group, and hinder personal adjustment to aging. Gerontology education therefore encourages students to examine their own feelings about aging, to gain a better understanding of reality through closer contact with older persons, and to develop a more positive perception of many older persons. The Syracuse University *Instructor's Handbook for the Development of a Basic Course in Gerontology* emphasizes this aspect of instruction, as does Hartford (1978) in her description of the goals of the University of Southern California degree program.

Several studies have attempted to measure the change in attitude toward older people that results from exposure to educational experiences. For instance, Cicchetti et al. (1973) reported that a course on aging within a school of medicine had as one of its objectives the improvement of attitudes toward older people. Their evaluation indicated that negative attitudes remained prevalent even after the completion of the course. Hudis (1974) likewise had as her primary goal the modification of negative attitudes toward older people. She found that there was some positive attitude change. Although other researchers have reported similarly weak changes, the affective elements of gerontology instruction are of substantial importance to many instructors and are likely to continue to be one of the major purposes of gerontology education.

The fourth purpose listed previously for academic gerontology courses is the development of the skills to analyze research findings in the field, to help students develop their capabilities to think and write, and to understand the difficulties involved in studying populations of older people. These objectives go beyond the utility of gerontology knowledge for the individual; they use gerontology content as a medium to teach the skills of a disciplined mind, those which have been common in liberal education for centuries (Schonfield and Chatfield, 1976).

## Gerontology as a Profession

Although many writers have chosen to present gerontology as either a discipline, an interdisciplinary area, or an academic pursuit, a large portion of the gerontology education literature views gerontology as a developing field of professional service. The need for increased instruction is based upon the premise that new community and institutional services will require well-prepared manpower, and instructional programs are primarily designed to teach the skills needed for service delivery, planning, community organization, administration, and evaluation.

Professional skills are advocated for graduate level instruction with students expected to learn therapeutic intervention or research skills that could be used in a variety of settings. Since professional service is provided to older people by a wide variety of agencies and institutions and by a large number of professional groups, the skills students are expected to acquire are likely to vary significantly from one educational program to the next. At the newly developed School of Gerontology at the University of Southern California, students are expected to obtain knowledge of individual and group methods, program planning and administration, community development, and research utilization (Hartford, 1978).

Other authors suggest that students develop skills in a clinical setting (Harbaugh, 1976) or that they be prepared to develop and administer community-based services (Fauri, 1974). In many programs today the student's interest in employment is very high, and the providing of salable skills is a top priority. There seems to be relatively little specificity in the literature on what these skills should be; most writers appear to set their priorities from the standpoint of their own professional or disciplinary background and to see the gerontology graduate as having skills similar to those of other human service professionals. Thus, Hartford's list of skills parallels those of social work—her profession of origin.

An adjunct to many professional practice skills is the preparation and encouragement of the prospective practitioner to become a social advocate. Hess (1976) has pointed out that much gerontology research is undertaken as a means to affect public policy or practice in the human service professions. There appears to be a deep strain of moral indignation in gerontologists which encourages the critical/confrontative approach to solving the problems of older people. Educational programs seem to have a similar emphasis. They advocate improved quality of life for older people as a primary goal and encourage students to take aggressive action to assure that this goal is achieved. Political activity is viewed as the most viable approach to this problem, and students are instructed in planning and organizing strategies for community improvement.

This doctrine of advocacy carries over into the evangelical fervor of many faculty members. In addition to community and political activities for the betterment of older people, faculty members have set as a personal as well as organizational goal the gerontologizing of the institution of higher education. This is done by encouraging other faculty to engage in gerontology instruction, research, and service. The goal is to spread the influence into as many academic and professional units as possible, encouraging faculty to expand their interest to such an extent that every undergraduate is exposed to some gerontology course work (Kaplan, 1978). This zeal for expansion is witnessed in a few other academic areas but is an explicit aim of many in gerontology.

The expansionist emphasis explains the strong theme in the literature regarding the need for trained manpower to conduct community and institutional services effectively for older people. The literature has lamented the fact that so few persons are presently available to accept employment in the field (Birren, Woodruff, and Bergman, 1972; Donahue, 1970; Birren, 1971; Woodruff and Birren, 1974). Data on manpower needs have typically been generated from projected growth of agencies and institutions such as nursing homes, senior centers, home health care programs, homes for the aged, transportation services, nutrition programs, and government agencies. Often, these projections have been based more on hope than on any valid formula for estimating program growth.

The major piece of work in this area was the report sponsored by the Administration on Aging on *Manpower Supply and Demand in Aging and Training Programs and Training Needs* (1968). This study compiled the projections for future manpower needs in several gerontologically related professional and practice areas. Although it was based entirely on secondary data analysis, these figures have been quoted in many contexts and have gained wide acceptance as real measures of future employment expectations.

The Administration on Aging in cooperation with the Bureau of Labor Statistics has embarked on a project with the potential to improve the quality of available manpower data. These two agencies are publishing a series of occasional papers on manpower needs which examine various occupational categories and institutional requirements. The first of these papers, published in 1976, provided an overview of the nursing home industry and indicated that the number of personnel needed would nearly double between 1973 and 1985 (*AoA Occasional Papers in Gerontology*, 1976). A breakdown by job category provides a great deal of insight into the type of future employees who will be most in demand.

Although the number of jobs continues to grow, many potential areas are limited by severe financial restrictions. Often there is a major discrepancy between need for personnel and available financial resources. For instance, nursing homes could provide considerably better patient care and rehabilitative services if they could expand their professional nursing and therapeutic staff. Unfortunately, they are typically unable to absorb the increased costs that would result; the manpower need exists, but jobs do not. This situation is evident in the historical imbalance between gerontology graduates and jobs in this field. For a time in the early 1970s, there were more gerontology graduates than jobs. As increased government funding for community programs and institutional care has become available, the demand for qualified personnel has increased and opportunities for gerontology graduates have expanded so that there is currently a shortage of well-educated professionals in many areas.

The employment situation for gerontology graduates is far from resolved, however. Most of the jobs have traditionally fallen into other professional service categories—nursing, administration, social work, recreation, counseling, or community organization—and are often filled by graduates from these areas. The *Occupational Outlook Quarterly* (1976) recently published a whole issue on gerontologically related employment which provides a good overview of the types and levels of positions available. Unfortunately, even this does not resolve the questions about the skills and knowledge needed in this employment or the most effective ways to prepare personnel for professional service in the field of aging.

## Conclusions

The literature of gerontology education reveals the problems facing the area and the progress made in the past 20 years. It is primarily descriptive, emphasizing current program operation with initial attempts to identify and clarify the purposes and outcomes of gerontology education.

There have been several different emphases in the literature, often contradicting each other. There is an interest in developing gerontology as a discipline that will draw upon but remain apart from other academic and professional units of higher education. At the same time there is much support for the view that gerontology should be incorporated into the traditional disciplines and professions as an interest area.

Some writers have viewed gerontology education as an academic undertaking that can provide students with an understanding of human growth, personal adjustment, and intellectual inquiry. Other writers have chosen the point of view that gerontology is more appropriately viewed as a social problem and service area, with the preparation of practitioners a desired outcome.

There is little consistency or agreement in the field at the present time. Some observers applaud this situation, saying that a period of searching will be necessary before the broad outlines of the field are clarified (Seltzer, 1974; Beattie, 1978). Others suggest that a developmental process is at work in which gerontology education structures are planted within existing departments, later to bloom as autonomous and separate entities (Peterson, 1978a). It is appropriate to formulate an initial statement on the nature and purpose of the field. No final or definitive statement can be made at this time, for the future doubtless holds many changes; however, the following chapters are an attempt to begin the process of analysis in order to clarify and define the issues that have been identified in the literature (Weg, 1974; Linn and Carmichael, 1974) but have yet to be resolved.

## References

Atchley, Robert C., and Mildred M. Seltzer. *Developing Educational Programs in the Field of Aging*. Oxford, Ohio: Scripps Foundation Gerontology Center, Miami University, no date.

*AoA Occasional Papers in Gerontology: Manpower Needs in the Field of Aging: The Nursing Home Industry*. Washington, D.C.: National Clearinghouse on Aging, USDHEW, 1976.

Baumhover, Lorin A. Toward the Development of Certification Programs in Gerontology. In Seltzer, Mildred M., Harvey Sterns, and Tom Hickey (eds.). *Gerontology in Higher Education: Perspectives and Issues*. Belmont, Calif.: Wadsworth Publishing, 1978.

Beattie, Walter M., Jr. Gerontology Curricula: Multidisciplinary Frameworks, Interdisciplinary Structures and Disciplinary Depth. *The Gerontologist*, 1974, *14*, 545–549.

Beattie, Walter M., Jr. Major Concerns and Future Directions in Gerontology and Higher Education. In Seltzer, Mildred M., Harvey Sterns, and Tom Hickey (eds.). *Gerontology in Higher Education: Perspectives and Issues*. Belmont, Calif.: Wadsworth Publishing, 1978.

Birren, James E. *Training in Aging: Background and Issues*. Washington, D.C.: White House Conference on Aging, 1971.

Birren, James E., and Diana S. Woodruff. Academic and Professional Training in the Psychology of Aging. In Eisdorfer, Carl, and M. Powell Lawton (eds.). *The Psychology of Adult Development and Aging*. Washington, D.C.: The American Psychological Association, 1973.

Birren, James E., Diana S. Woodruff, and Simon Bergman. Research, Demonstration and Training: Issues and Methodologies in Social Gerontology. *The Gerontologist*, 1972, *12*, 49–83.

Chebotarev, D. F. Importance of Research in Gerontology for Education and Training in Geriatrics. *Educational Gerontology: An International Quarterly*, 1976, *1*, 199–203.

Cicchetti, Domenic V., C. Richard Flethcher, Emanuel Lehner, and Jules V. Coleman. Effects of a Social Medicine Course on the Attitudes of Medical Students Toward the Elderly: A Controlled Study. *Journal of Gerontology*, 1973, *28*, 370–373.

Cohen, Cyril. Techniques in Teaching Geriatric Medicine. In Anderson, W. Ferguson, and T. G. Judge (eds.). *Geriatric Medicine*. New York: Academic Press, 1974.

Cohen, Ruth G. Graduate Social Work Training in a Multipurpose Geriatric Center. *The Gerontologist*, Winter 1971, *11*, 352–355.

Cooney, Cyprian J. Functions of Academic Gerontology (Undergraduate Level). In Seltzer, Mildred M., Harvey Sterns, and Tom Hickey (eds.). *Gerontology in Higher Education: Perspectives and Issues*. Belmont, Calif.: Wadsworth Publishing, 1978.

Donahue, Wilma. Recruiting and Training of Personnel Required by the Organization of Gerontology. *First International Course in Gerontology*. Paris: International Center of Social Gerontology, 1970.

Donahue, Wilma. Training in Social Gerontology. *Geriatrics*, 1960, *15*, 801–809.

Ehrlich, Ira F., and Phyllis D. Ehrlich. A Four-part Framework to Meet the Responsibilities of Higher Education to Gerontology. *Educational Gerontology: An International Quarterly*, July-Sept. 1976, *1*, 251–260.

Elias, Merrill F. Postdoctoral Research Training in Aging: Interdisciplinary or Unidisciplinary. Paper presented at the 25th Annual Meeting of the Gerontological Society, San Juan, Puerto Rico, December 1972.

Fauri, David P. Guest Editorial: Educating for Gerontological Leadership Roles. *The Gerontologist*, 1974, *14*, 466.

Freeman, Joseph T. A Survey of Geriatric Education: Catalogues of United States Medical Schools. *Journal of the American Geriatrics Society*, 1971, *19*, 746–762.

Goldman, Ralph. Geriatrics as a Specialty: Problems and Prospects. *The Gerontologist*, 1974, *14*, 468–471.

Gunter, Laurie M. and Carmen A. Estes. *Education for Gerontic Nursing.* New York: Springer, 1978.

Harbaugh, Joseph D. Clinical Training and Legal Services for Older People: The Role of the Law Schools. *The Gerontologist*, 1976, *16*, 447–452.

Harris, Raymond. Model for a Graduate Geriatric Program at a University Medical School. *The Gerontologist*, 1975, *15*, 304–307.

Hartford, Margaret E. Career Education for the Preparation of Practitioners ✓ in Gerontology with Special Reference to Adult Educators. In Sherron, Ronald H., and D. Barry Lumsden (eds.). *Introduction to Educational Gerontology*. Washington D.C.: Hemisphere Publishing, 1978.

Hess, Beth B. Introduction to the Use of Social Gerontology. In Hess, Beth  *check* B. (ed.). *Growing Old in America*. New Brunswick, N.J.: Transaction Books, 1976.

Hudis, Ann. An Introductory Course in Gerontology: Development and ? Evaluation. *The Gerontologist*, 1974, *14*, 312–315.

Hulicka, Irene M., and John B. Morganti. An Undergraduate Concentration in the Psychology of Aging: Approach, Program and Evaluation. *Educational Gerontology: An International Quarterly*, 1976, *1*, 107–118.

*Instructor's Handbook for the Development of a Basic Course in Gerontology, An.* Syracuse, N.Y.: Syracuse University All-University Gerontology Center, 1975.

Johnston, James O. Social Workers Needs for Education. In Anderson, W. Ferguson, and T. G. Judge (eds.). *Geriatric Medicine*. New York: Academic Press, 1974.

Kaplan, Jerome. The Effect of Extension of Life on Undergraduate Academic Gerontology. In Seltzer, Mildred M., Harvey Sterns, and Tom Hickey (eds.). *Gerontology in Higher Education: Perspectives and Issues*. Belmont, Calif.: Wadsworth Publishing, 1978. *incl.*

Kleemeier, Robert W. Gerontology as a Discipline. *The Gerontologist*, 1965, *shortage of* 5, 237–239. *trained manpower*

Koller, Marvin R. *Social Gerontology*. New York: Random House, 1968.

Linn, Margaret W., and Lynn P. Carmichael. Introducing Pre-professionals ✗ to Gerontology. *The Gerontologist*, 1974, *14*, 476–478.

Lowy, Louis, and Leo Miller. Guest Editorial: Toward Greater Movement for Gerontology in Social Work Education. *The Gerontologist*, 1974, *14*, 466–467.

*Manpower Supply and Demand in Aging and Training Programs and* ✓ *Training Needs*. Washington, D.C.: Surveys and Research Corporation, 1968.

McCall, Janet. Education in Geriatric Nursing. In Anderson, W. Ferguson, and T. G. Judge (eds.). *Geriatric Medicine*. New York: Academic Press, 1974.

Moberg, David O. Needs Felt by the Clergy for Ministries to the Aging. *The Gerontologist* , 1975, *15*, 170–175.

*Occupational Outlook Quarterly*. Special Issue: Working with Older People. Washington, D.C.: Bureau of Labor Statistics, U.S. Department of Labor, Fall 1976, *20*.

Peterson, David A. Educational Gerontology: The State of the Art. *Educational Gerontology: An International Quarterly*, 1976, *1*, 61–73.

Peterson, David A. An Overview of Gerontology Education. In Seltzer, Mildred M., Harvey Sterns, and Tom Hickey (eds.). *Gerontology in Higher Education: Perspectives and Issues*. Belmont, Calif.: Wadsworth Publishing, 1978a.

Peterson, David A. Toward a Definition of Educational Gerontology. In Lumsden, Barry S., and Ronald Sherron (eds.). *Introduction to Educational Gerontology*. Washington D.C.: Hemisphere Publishing, 1978b.

Rodstein, Manuel. A Model Curriculum for an Elective Course in Geriatrics. *The Gerontologist*, 1973, *13*, 231–235.

Safier, Gwendolyn. Undergraduate Nursing Students and Their Experience in Gerontology. *The Gerontologist*, 1975, *15*, 165–169.

Schonfield, David, and Sally Chatfield. Goals, Purposes, and Future of Undergraduate Education in the Psychology of Aging. *Educational Gerontology: An International Quarterly*, 1976, *1*, 391–397.

Seltzer, Mildred M. Education in Gerontology: An Evolutionary Analogy. *The Gerontologist*, 1974, *14*, 308–311.

Tibbitts, Clark. Origin, Scope and Fields of Social Gerontology. In Tibbitts, Clark (ed.). *Handbook of Social Gerontology*. Chicago: University of Chicago Press, 1960.

Tibbitts, Clark. Social Gerontology in Education for the Professions. In Kushner, Rose, and Marion E. Bunch (eds.). *Graduate Education in Aging within the Social Sciences*. Ann Arbor, Mich.: Division of Gerontology, University of Michigan, 1967.

Weg, Ruth B. Response: A View from Curricula for Gerontology. *The Gerontologist*, 1974, *14*, 549–553.

Woodruff, Diana S., and James E. Birren. Training for the Professionals in the Field of Aging: Needs, Goals, Models, and Means. In Schwartz, Arthur N., and Ivan N. Mensh (eds.). *Professional Obligations and Approaches to the Aged*. Springfield, Ill.: Charles C Thomas, 1974.

# 4

# Issues in Gerontology Education

The prevailing issues in gerontology education, like those in many arenas of higher education, rest upon the question of *goals.* The goals of higher education, including those of gerontology education, embody the philosophical underpinnings for the missions, objectives, purposes, and functions of instructional programs. Goals are often amorphous philosophical ideals espoused by institutions but never fully understood by even the most sophisticated educators. Therefore, for clarity, in this chapter goals will be defined as ideals that guide the development of specific program functions, missions, and educational outcomes.

Philosophers and students of higher education have suggested that the primary goal of American post-secondary education is learning. With this goal representing the ultimate result of the research, service, and teaching mission of higher education, all other goals become secondary correlates, undertaken to achieve this one overriding concern.

Historically, the goals for higher education of character building and acculturation have predominated. One example of this view comes from Robert Maynard Hutchins (1936), who, during his presidency at the University of Chicago, asserted: "Our purpose is to turn out well-tubbed young Americans who know how to behave in the American environment" (pp. 28–29). While this characterization of well-schooled youth may invoke nostalgic reminiscence of our goals prior to the post–World War II technological revolution, more practical and complex goals now pervade higher education. Present-day educators reflect the dichotomy of modern goals for higher education. Writers such as Brubacher (1977), Mayhew (1969), and Henderson and Henderson (1975) have summarized the evolution of educational philosophy from the liberal education traditions of early universities through the advent of research universities such as Johns Hopkins, Harvard Graduate School, and the University of Michigan to the era of vocationalism, whose institutional prototypes are junior and community colleges and professional schools. There remain many small, often church-related colleges that attempt to follow the character-building model espoused by Hutchins, but these institutions represent goals that are at best anachronistic. For the majority of institutions, as well as for students, who must be attracted if any school is to survive, there is the belief that some balance between the romantic ideals of whole-man education and the consumer-based realities of professional education is the sought-after goal.

While goal statements provide a vague understanding of the directions and ends of higher education institutions, a far more useful though less lofty and general statement can be derived from examining the "purposes" of higher education. Purposes "refer to stated conceptions of the mission of systems, groups, or types of colleges. Thus, we can speak of the purposes of American higher education, the liberal arts college, or the California community colleges" (Peterson, 1970, p.3). In this way, we can move from the broad philosophically based goals for institutions to the purposes of their various components. Purposes, because more specific than goals, are often the only guidelines available for the program development and review processes.

The purpose statement developed by the University of Wisconsin Faculty Interdisciplinary Studies Committee on the Future of Man (Potter et al., 1970) proposed that, "The primary purpose of the University is to provide an environment in which faculty and students can discover, examine critically, preserve, and transmit the knowledge, wisdom, and values that will help ensure the survival of the present and future generations with improvement in the quality of life." This statement presents the end (learning) as well as the reason for that end (improved quality of life) in such a manner that today's "multiversities" may pursue the same goals through a variety of means.

Objectives are the most specific statement of desired outcome for institutions of higher education. Objectives, more definable and measurable than purposes or goals, usually include a time frame in which the objective is to be achieved. Objectives are generally quite specific and provide a guide for the particular activities to be undertaken.

## Issues in Gerontology Education

The determination of goals, purposes, and objectives in higher education can be viewed as a process of exclusion. Rather than attempting to undertake all available avenues to facilitate learning, limited resources require that some approaches be chosen over others. Thus, dichotomies tend to develop around the basic choices of higher education. This has been true of gerontology education as it is of all instruction. The potential program outcomes are identified and the differing results are compared with each other as well as with the goal, which is ultimately the guide to rational decision making.

The three major issues of purpose currently facing gerontology education are as follows:

1. Should gerontology be taught in breadth (broad-based, general education) or in depth (narrowly focused specialized education)?

2. Should gerontology be organized as a separate, distinct field of study (discipline or profession) or as an ancillary specialty connected with established scientific or professional fields (multidisciplinary)?

3. Should gerontology teach skills and knowledge that relate to practice in an occupational role (profession) or knowledge and attitude, which may lead toward understanding and appreciation (academic)?

Thus, the three issues deal with three separate categories of purpose: content (breadth vs. depth), organization (distinct field vs. ancillary specialization), and use of the education (professional practice vs. liberal knowledge).

These three substantive issues may be considered as independent dichotomies in the abstract, but in reality they are two ends of a continuum; purposes may be chosen in the middle rather than on one end. Moreover, the three issues overlap to such a degree that it is often impossible to discuss one without considering another.

### Breadth versus Depth

The dilemma of specialization versus general education (breadth vs. depth) is a phenomenon of recent history. The "knowledge explosion" has produced vast amounts of information in practically every discipline. It is no longer possible for the "Renaissance Man" to be a veritable encyclopedia of all knowledge. The age of the specialist has come and only a few dedicated scholars are able to master the elements of even one burgeoning disciplinary specialty.

This enormous increase in information is responsible for the creation of numerous academic and professional departments and schools and has wrought distinct changes in the college and university curriculum. According to Henderson and Henderson (1975), the breadth of education has continually diminished while specialized education has grown proportionately larger. Departmentalization brought about by the increase of knowledge has made it increasingly difficult for faculties to offer students thorough preparation in one area as well as exposure to the broad scope of human knowledge.

When facing these issues from the standpoint of gerontology education, the question is whether instruction should lead to a broad understanding of conceptual and empirical knowledge available from several disciplinary and practical perspectives or whether more concentrated knowledge of the methods and content of one problem orientation is appropriate. Since gerontology is generally assumed to draw both its methods and content from the traditional disciplines and professional fields, a broad awareness of the field would include some understanding of the biological, physiological, psychological, behavioral, sociological, philosophical, religious, economic, political, legal, medical, and mental health areas as well as an understanding of contemporary services, agencies, and personnel who are concerned about older people. Obviously, gaining such a breadth of knowledge would prohibit the individual student from achieving great depth in any area.

On the other hand, the instructional program could easily be designed so that the student could learn a great deal about one area —for example, the mental functions of old age—along with the assessment tools, intervention strategies, and agencies and institutions relevant to that area. This would provide sufficient depth to claim extensive knowledge in the area or to undertake research or practice, depending upon personal inclinations and available opportunities.

In considering undergraduate education in gerontology, the issue is not particularly difficult, nor contested. The bulk of undergraduate programs, whether in a junior or community college, a four-year college, or a multiversity, subscribe to the notion of general education with a distribution of electives and requirements that allows for breadth of content exposure. This arrangement easily allows for a minor concentration in areas like gerontology. Even those institutions that offer a specialized degree in gerontology at the undergraduate level most often are providing merely a major concentration in the field rather than a highly specialized, narrowly and deeply focused curriculum.

The issue becomes more complex, however, when we examine graduate education in gerontology. There are several instances of colleges and universities that now offer a master's degree representing a more sophisticated level of specialization in gerontology. In fact, in isolated instances, some institutions have proposed the development of a Ph.D. or an applied doctorate specifically directed toward gerontological studies.

The purpose of this graduate education in gerontology has not been consistent among the various institutions involved. Three possible outcomes can be identified, but only two seem common at this time. Some, such as North Texas State University, provide intensive preparation for persons who plan to administer nursing homes or homes for the aged. Others, such as the University of South Florida, emphasize planning and delivery of human services. These two programs suggest that gerontology has achieved a level of knowledge and skill equivalent to other professional fields and that preparation in depth for practice is the purpose of the program.

On the other hand, it would be possible to offer a master's degree in gerontology which would prepare a person to enter a doctoral program. Thus, depth in concepts and research would be emphasized more than skills for practice. To date, few colleges or universities seem inclined to undertake this type of education. Since doctoral degrees in gerontology are not available, such preparation is inappropriate at this time.

A third approach is to provide a general overview of the field. Students are offered some exposure to various fields related to gerontology without gaining either skills for practice or depth of understanding. It would appear that these programs provide general exposure to gerontology at an academic level, a purpose not typically cited as an intended outcome of graduate instruction. For individual courses, this is often the stated purpose, but for graduate degree programs, the preparation for practice seems to be the more appropriate outcome.

Graduate instruction in gerontology does not often lead to a degree but may be taken as an emphasis or specialty area in connection with a disciplinary or professional degree. If the study is part of a master's degree in a discipline such as psychology or sociology, then the purpose of the instruction might well be to develop academic depth. This is a reasonable purpose and one which is typical of much graduate instruction in gerontology today.

The issue of depth versus breadth then, although not resolved in practice, would seem to be best decided by the level of instruction. At the undergraduate level, breadth seems most appropriate and is, in fact, the norm. At the graduate level, depth is a more defensible purpose, but some current programs have chosen to offer a broad education, which is questionable at best. Many programs have chosen a practice-oriented degree while others have chosen academic education as an adjunct to a disciplinary degree.

## Distinct Field versus Ancillary Field

If gerontology is to be given the organizational structure accorded to the traditional disciplines, it must merit similar criteria. Dressel and Mayhew (1974) provide a definition of a discipline which indicates the attributes to be met in order to meet disciplinary expectations: (1) a general body of knowledge, which can be, at worst, forced into some reasonably logical taxonomy; (2) a specialized vocabulary and a generally accepted basic literature; (3) some generally accepted body of theory and some generally understood techniques for theory testing and revision; (4) a generally agreed-upon methodology; and (5) recognized techniques for replication and revalidation of research and scholarship. Whether gerontology can claim disciplinary status based upon these criteria is subject to considerable doubt. Although some gerontology educators believe that if gerontology does not yet possess these characteristics, it soon will, most others would agree that it does not, cannot, and should not.

The major difficulty with attempting to recognize gerontology as a discipline is the recentness of its development and the rapidity of its expansion within higher education. Proponents for disciplinary status often argue that gerontology must seek this status in order to survive the current retrenchment in higher education. Legitimization based upon a departmental designation with the concomitant ability to award degrees has provided strong motivation in many recent attempts to attain disciplinary recognition. These attempts, however, are based upon organizational survival rather than a belief in the correctness of the disciplinary classification. It would seem more appropriate, although slower, to accept criteria such as those presented previously and build the necessary logically based arguments for testing gerontology's strength as an emerging discipline. The *Handbooks on Aging* are a step toward developing a taxonomy and basic literature, but theory and methodology remain to be expanded, and few persuasive arguments have been presented on the validity of viewing gerontology as a discipline.

The other alternative in developing a distinct field of gerontology is to argue that gerontology is a profession and that the appropriate organizational structure should resemble those of such professional or practice areas as social work, public administration, or nursing. In order to become a profession it would be necessary for gerontology to meet certain generally accepted criteria. Greenwood (1976) suggests that a profession has five clear and accepted attributes: (1) a systematic body of theory that directs professional practice; (2) professional authority that allows for a monopoly on the provision of the particular service; (3) community support and sanction of the authority of the members of the profession; (4) a code of ethics that directs practice; and (5) a professional culture, which includes agencies and institutions, educational programs, and formal organizations for members of the profession.

At the present time it is difficult to assert that gerontology is a profession. There is little clarity on the type of professional service that is provided; there is no professional authority, no community sanction, and no ethical code. It is not improbable, however, that the coming years will witness movement toward a profession as more education programs are created and graduates seek jobs in the human service areas. There remain many unanswered questions about the type and level of service that should be provided and the relationship of the practicing gerontologist to other professionals who also offer services to older people.

A few attempts to define at least a part of the profession of gerontology are currently underway. These are typically within educational institutions instructing graduate students in some aspect of the field such as human service delivery or housing management. There is little work currently being done, however, to clarify the roles of gerontology practitioners or to determine the knowledge and skills that will be most useful in carrying out the defined role.

The opposite point of view is that gerontology is not a discipline or a profession but is an adjunct to the established disciplines or professions. This position is based upon the belief that gerontology is a composite of methodologies, theories, and practice representing a multidisciplinary approach that is not sufficiently mature or unique to stand alone. This view is supported by the fact that many pioneer programs of instruction in gerontology, which now have established themselves, adopted a multidisciplinary focus. As new instructional undertakings were initiated at other colleges and universities, these mature programs have provided advice encouraging others to accept this arrangement as the most appropriate at present.

Multidisciplinary (or transdisciplinary or interdisciplinary) programs, which derive concepts and ideas from more than one discipline (Dressel, 1976), isolate those elements common to several disciplines in relation to a major focus for study—in this case human aging. A discipline, on the other hand, is taught, studied, and discussed for purposes of mastery of content rather than for consideration of applications.

Applying these guidelines to the field of gerontology provides some measure of clarity. If gerontology is to be thought of as a content area worthy of study and continuing research for the sake of disciplinary development, then the argument for disciplinary classification holds. However, it would appear that in most programs of gerontology education across the country, the prevailing emphasis is on the development of practical competencies rather than the pursuit of scientific truths. This position would suggest that the multidisciplinary approach is most appropriate for gerontology. For, as Dressel (1976) says, "Unless the focus of a course is on a problem, concept, or concern which transcends the disciplines, it is difficult to achieve a meaningful interdisciplinary stance. Indeed, the only way to be truly independent of disciplinary boundaries is to deal with issues that are supradisciplinary. The disciplines then become—as they should—reservoirs of organized knowledge and modes of search" (p. 300).

In applying this concept to the organizational structures that exist in gerontology education, several distinct possibilities present themselves. Some educational institutions have chosen to create an interdisciplinary committee to organize gerontology instruction. Others have a coordinating group of faculty who meet regularly, with instruction done in individual departments. Elsewhere some instruction is done in departments and some in a gerontology unit, which is a gap-filling, supplemental organization. In short, the issue of gerontology structure is not one easily resolved.

## Academic versus Professional Education

Should preparation for work in the field of gerontology be seen as a career-related group of specialties requiring training experiences focused on particular aspects of practice for a specific occupational role, or has gerontology accumulated sufficient theoretical and scientific depth for gerontology education to focus on liberalizing the disciplines, considering aging in relation to science, the arts, the humanities, etc.? This issue, like the others, is not unique to gerontology; scholars in higher education have attempted to deal with it for many years.

Upon closer consideration it appears that further clarification of terms is needed. *Professional education* connotes educating persons for occupations that deal with the problems and concerns of the aging. *Academic* has two possible meanings: discipline-based search for knowledge and truth; or a liberal arts/general education point of view. The latter is most appropriate here.

Brubacher (1977) poses the issue in the form of two questions.

> Should it [higher education] consist of general education, a modest and less than Baconian survey of the higher learning, leaving specialization to graduate and professional education? Or should general education share the undergraduate curriculum with specialized, especially career-motivated, education? [pp. 68–69].

This statement emphasizes the distinction between undergraduate and graduate/professional levels of higher education, but does not resolve the issue. Is there an appropriate modal position for all gerontology education, or will it be necessary to specify different outcomes for undergraduate general education, for professional instruction, and for academic graduate education?

Many current undergraduate programs suggest that students in the Associate's and Bachelor's degree programs are being prepared to perform professional and paraprofessional roles. There are graduate programs with both an emphasis in academic (scientific) preparation and in professional preparation. There is not at this time, however, a clear explication of the distinct and different outcomes for these different types of instruction.

At the graduate level the same issue of professional versus academic outcomes exists. Although the field of gerontology does not currently meet the criteria for a profession, much instruction is oriented toward preparing individuals for a practice role. There are expectations that the field of service will be clarified and strengthened in the future.

In the academic area, two emphases may be developed. First, it is possible to view gerontology as a discipline, although gerontology does not now nor is it likely in the near future to meet the criteria of a discipline, and to prepare persons for research and teaching

within that discipline. Second, gerontology education may emphasize the general or liberal aspects of education, providing students
with an understanding of content showing some of the attitude components of the aging process.

Critics of the professional school and academic discipline approach to graduate education in gerontology suggest that there is
insufficient theoretical uniqueness in gerontology to allow deep and
narrow studies at the post-baccalaureate level; nor is there a recognized professional role for "gerontologists" which justifies development of professional education programs in aging.

On the other hand, critics of the liberal education approach
suggest that although this is appropriate for an undergraduate degree, it offers neither the depth nor the skills that should accompany
the graduate degree education. Thus, there is little consensus on the
most appropriate purposes for gerontology education.

## Conclusions

Three major issues confront gerontology education today. These are:
breadth versus depth; gerontology as a distinct field versus an adjunct to a traditional field; and professional versus academic preparation. Although these issues have been treated as separate concerns,
the interrelationships among them are great, and they may be combined to form a matrix of purposes for gerontology education. By
selecting one of the dichotomies for each of the three issues, the
observer of gerontology education can identify eight possible combinations of purposes for gerontology education:
  1. Breadth, distinct field, professional
  2. Breadth, distinct field, academic
  3. Breadth, ancillary field, professional
  4. Breadth, ancillary field, academic
  5. Depth, distinct field, professional
  6. Depth, distinct field, academic
  7. Depth, ancillary field, professional
  8. Depth, ancillary field, academic
These eight choices may be described in terms of the type and
level of instruction most appropriate. For instance, choice 8, depth,
ancillary field, and academic orientation, is appropriate at the graduate level for a specialization in gerontology in connection with a
degree in a disciplinary field (psychology, for instance). This arrange-

ment would be consistent with the thinking of many persons in the field and would be a most appropriate combination of purposes, especially at the doctoral level.

Choice 7, depth, ancillary field, and professional orientation, is a combination widely used today. In this instance gerontology education would be provided in the skills that professionals such as social workers or counselors need in order to serve older people. The instruction would not lead to a degree in gerontology but would more likely relate to the professional degree in another area, with gerontology being an ancillary area of instruction.

Choice 6, depth, distinct field, and academic orientation, suggests that gerontology is a discipline and should be taught as a doctoral program. This is generally considered an inappropriate combination of purposes.

Choice 5, depth, distinct field, and professional orientation, is appropriate to a professional degree in gerontology. This is probably most valuable at the graduate level and is likely to become more common in the future as additional degree programs in gerontology are developed.

Choice 4, breadth, ancillary field, and academic perspective, is appropriate to undergraduate specializations in connection with degrees in one of the disciplinary areas. Since breadth is most appropriate at the undergraduate level, the academic emphasis allows for a degree program that includes knowledge and attitude in many of the traditional areas leading toward specialization in graduate school or toward a liberal education designed as preparation for life.

Choice 3, breadth, ancillary field, and professional orientation, is appropriate for an undergraduate program to prepare students for entry-level professional service in one of the established professions —social work, education, nursing, etc. This combination of purposes emphasizes the liberal background of breadth while providing some of the skills needed for practice.

Choice 2, breadth, distinct field, and academic orientation, is appropriate for an undergraduate degree in gerontology. This would provide a broad exposure to various fields and would culminate in a degree in gerontology. This would not be a practice orientation but rather an understanding of the concepts and data of the field so that a liberal education could be gained.

Choice 1, breadth, distinct field, and professional orientation, would result in a general knowledge of gerontology but with a degree aimed toward professional practice. This is the type of educational experience that is being offered by a number of colleges and universities, but it does not seem to be appropriate since by definition it will fail to be either professional or broad.

The point of this analysis is not so much to suggest that one purpose is better than another, but that a combination of purposes will lead to more or less positive outcomes for gerontology education. The purposes are all valuable, but they are not all attainable in a single program which must operate with limited resources, limited staff, and limited time. This analysis should make it possible to determine which programs have a reasonable chance of meeting their stated purposes and which are likely to fail.

## References

Brubacher, J.S. *On The Philosophy of Higher Education*. San Francisco: Jossey-Bass, 1977.

Dressel, P.L. *Handbook of Academic Evaluation*. San Francisco: Jossey-Bass, 1976.

Dressel, P.L., and L.B. Mayhew. *Higher Education as a Field of Study*. San Francisco: Jossey-Bass, 1974.

Greenwood, Ernest. Attributes of a Profession. In Gilbert, Neil, and Harry Specht (eds.). *The Emergence of Social Welfare and Social Work*. Itasca, Ill.: F.E. Peacock Publishers, 1976.

Henderson, A.D., and J.G. Henderson. *Higher Education in America*. San Francisco: Jossey-Bass, 1975.

Hutchins, R.M. *The Higher Learning in America*. New Haven: Yale University Press, 1936.

Mayhew, L.B. *Colleges Today and Tomorrow*. San Francisco: Jossey-Bass, 1969.

Peterson, R.E. *The Crisis of Purpose: Definition and Uses of Institutional Goals*. Washington, D.C.: ERIC Clearinghouse on Higher Education, The George Washington University, 1970.

Potter, V.R., et al. Purpose and Function of the University, *Science*, No. 168, March, 1970.

# 5

# The Outcomes of Gerontology Education

The purposes of gerontology education set forth in the preceding chapter form the basis for specifying a series of outcomes that may result from undergraduate and graduate instruction in gerontology. These outcomes, defined as the products of higher education, are measurable and/or observable ends toward which educators strive in their teaching, research, and service. These ends require clarity and specificity so that the final results of the instruction can be adequately measured and defended.

Today, the majority of colleges, schools, and departments fail to develop well-conceived sets of purposes, thereby precluding the possibility of formulating measurable outcomes and often resulting in a disorganized, totally uncoordinated set of functions with little or no meaning. Activity on its own cannot be defended. It is progress toward some clearly articulated end which is required if the unit is to be accountable for its resources and staff.

Within the past ten years, roughly parallel to the accountability movement in higher education, educators have begun to explore specifications for measurable and observable outcomes. In one of the early volumes on the subject, Brown (1970) suggested a model in which outcomes of higher education could be specified and measured through the use of additive indexes. His recommendations were that outcomes be specified for the following categories: (1) Whole Man Growth; (2) Specialized Man Growth; (3) Growth of the "Pool of Knowledge"; (4) Growth of Society-at-Large; and (5) The Joy of Growing and Being in an Educational Environment. While these categories of outcomes indicate the major intents of higher education in general, it is very difficult to apply them to a specialized field of study such as gerontology.

Richman and Farmer (1974) provided an output taxonomy which is more in keeping with specific purposes and objectives. Their list includes:

1. Truth—a shorthand term for all types of searches for knowledge including faculty and student research activities,

2. Graduate students—the production of graduate degree holders in all fields,

3. Undergraduates—the production of undergraduates in all fields,

4. Security—protection, income, prestige, prerequisites, and academic freedom of professionals (faculty, major administrators, and some high-talent staff specialists) in the system,

5. Public service activities—including such items as faculty service, professional training, adult and extension education, summer programs, cultural events, and public use of facilities,

6. Research activities—both practical (applied) and theoretical (basic),

7. Cultural assimilation—the cultural development of staff and students,

8. Placement—jobs for students.

These outcomes suggest a broadly diverse set of activities to be undertaken in order to fulfill the functions of higher education. In most instances, however, academic units such as a gerontology education program would not be expected to fulfill the entire list, and in those areas where academic units were required to be accountable, for example in placement, the institution would provide considerable support.

Dressel and Mayhew (1974) suggest that the outcomes of higher education are best specified in the questions used in evaluating a given program. They suggest the following as a few of the pertinent questions guiding the evaluation of outcomes:

1. Are students satisfied with the program, with advising, and especially with internships?

2. Is there follow-up of graduates?

3. What is the quality of major writing assignments (papers, theses, dissertations, etc.)?

4. Is the faculty productive in research?

5. What is the range of service provided by the unit?

6. Are consultants used in program review?

7. Are students, faculty, and courses consistent with resources and goals?

8. What are the strengths and weaknesses as assessed by success in attaining goals?

While this list does not cover the entire spectrum of questions that can ascertain program outcomes, it is illustrative of the hard questions program faculty, administrators, and students must ask in maintaining the accountability of a particular program unit.

Micek, Service, and Lee (1975) provide some of the latest thinking on the results of higher education derived from the work of the Western Interstate Commission on Higher Education (WICHE). Their suggestions for the outcomes of higher education include:

1. *Student Growth and Development*—knowledge and skills development, educational career development, educational satisfaction, occupational career development, personal development, and social/cultural development,

2. *New Knowledge and Art Forms*—the development of research and creative activities which expand horizons regarding what is known, heard, and seen,

3. *Community Impact*—educational, service, and economic impact on the local area and on the nation.

These outcome specifications are the product of ten years of research on the development of comprehensive outcome specifications and measures. Although the WICHE outcomes investigations have resulted in the development of highly specific categorizations and measures, their utility is highly limited because of a lack of interest or understanding among the leaders in the higher education community.

The specification of outcomes for higher education, as with the specification of purposes, is of necessity broad based and general. Gerontology education outcomes do not always include all of those identified but will emphasize those based on the purposes appropriate for that unit. For example, a unit stressing the development of doctoral researchers would emphasize instruction on observable knowledge and skills that lead to methodological expertise. On the other hand, a program for the preparation of pre- or paraprofessionals for service occupations related to aging (e.g. geriatric nurse aide), would emphasize outcomes related to occupational training and service purposes.

The specification of outcomes for higher education has been given considerable attention in the literature. This focus is appropriate at present, when higher education institutions are faced with declining enrollments and serious questions about the relevance of a college degree. Gerontology educators, like their colleagues in other areas, will be well advised to formulate careful and precise outcome statements that permit the measurement of program progress toward stated purposes. In an attempt to assist the development of this undertaking, the following sections of this chapter describe three possible outcome categories for programs of gerontology education based upon the purposes described in Chapter 4.

## Outcomes for Gerontology Education

The outcomes we choose for gerontology education are closely related to our philosophical beliefs regarding what higher education should be. The fundamental philosophical orientations of a given educator will therefore be reflected in the characteristics of the program he or she leads. The Carnegie Commission on Higher Education (1973) suggested that there are three fundamental philosophical alternatives currently accepted in the United States: liberal education, scientific education, and professional education. The selection of one or a combination of these will generally determine the purposes and outcomes of gerontology education. Practically speaking there is little likelihood that any of the three alternatives exists in pure form. Since the advent of "Dewey-pragmatic" thought, American educators have evolved eclectic systems. These systems represent an amalgamation of several philosophical stances, oftentimes representing more of a cacophony of views than an organized pattern. The purposes discussed in Chapter 4 indicate, however, that it is possible to perceive the desired ultimate outcomes for gerontology education in nearly pure form while accepting eclectic inclinations.

## The Search for Values:
## Liberal Gerontology Education

In the strict sense, liberal gerontology education cannot be concerned with the development of the student in general education terms—"whole man growth" (Brown, 1970)—to the same extent that a college of liberal arts is. However, the educational philosophy will be the same and the specialized gerontology outcomes will be consistent with those of a liberal arts college. The ultimate student learning outcome would be the achievement of a broad-based understanding of the processes of aging, developed and promoted through the study of gerontological theory. Theoretical education is the heart of liberal education because it allows the enlargement of one's scope of action (Brubacher, 1977). Knowledge of the theoretical underpinnings of gerontology from the standpoint of the natural and social sciences and the humanities is one basic outcome of liberal gerontology education.

There is little or no place in liberal gerontology education for consideration of things practical. The emphasis is placed upon the development of appropriate attitudes and understandings requisite to knowing and understanding rather than doing. In this respect, the student-centered whole man growth outcomes for gerontology education must be highly coordinated with other components of the student's educational program, such as the outcomes associated with the major field of concentration. This consideration has many ramifications for the organization of studies, the orientation of faculty to the subject matter, the meaning of the credential awarded, and the direction given to the functions of research and public service.

*Organization of studies.* Students and faculty have a general education purpose in participating. The curriculum is organized and taught in a manner that reflects a value system devoid of practical outcomes, as defined by the terms *vocational* or *professional* education. Much of the curricular emphasis is placed on developing a broad and interdisciplinary conceptualization of the meaning of aging and the implications of that learning for the fate of mankind. The study of aging is viewed, not as a scientific or disciplinary endeavor, but as a mechanism to provide an overall perspective of man in the historical, philosophical, scientific, or social context under consideration.

The outcomes specified for liberal gerontology education are oriented toward breadth of knowledge in the academic sense. They would include students: (1) learning a broad, interdisciplinary overview of aging from the perspectives of the natural and social sciences; (2) developing the ability to conceptualize clearly from a theoretical point of view, with applications coming in experiential situations after graduation; and (3) demonstrating learning through scholarly activities (discussions, papers, etc.) which integrate the basic principles and lead toward new and unique explanations of selected aspects of aging. While problem centered in an academic sense, gerontology education would stress the mental agility necessary for discussion and problem solving of a theoretical/philosophical nature.

*Orientation of faculty to the subject matter.* Faculty employing a liberal education approach to gerontology prepare for instruction activities in an interdisciplinary manner. The faculty perceive of themselves as generalists in the field. Their orientation dictates that the subject matter of aging be taken from a whole man conceptual stance requiring that reading and writing assignments incorporate integration of theoretical principles rather than empirical explanations of physical or social data. Gerontology would be taught within a holistic framework, placing the emphasis on well-founded understandings of phenomena rather than on collecting and verifying discrete facts. The liberal gerontology educator approaches the subject matter of aging from the perspective of rigorous scholarship as this concept relates to the formulation of clearer meaning and integration with other knowledge relative to the understanding of the processes of aging. The orientation would be whole man growth in focus and function.

*Meaning of credentials.* Degrees or certificates awarded by programs espousing liberal gerontology education ideals mirror the credentials granted by liberal arts programs. In the case of a program offering a major in gerontology at the undergraduate level, the Bachelor of Arts is the standard degree. This degree has limited utility as an entry credential for a specified field of work. The meaning of a liberal education credential is that the student has successfully completed a comprehensive overview or survey of the processes of aging. This may result in an academic degree in gerontology or in a certificate, minor, or concentration in relation to a degree in a traditional discipline or occupational field. In the latter case, the student may gain some gerontology understanding while at the same time pursuing a job-oriented professional field. A liberal gerontology education credential, then, can be viewed as a corollary to the student's major; in that case, it supplements and enhances that major rather than conflicting with or supplanting it.

*Research.* Research, or in Brown's terms "growth of the pool of knowledge" (1970), within higher education is not restricted to specialized faculty with established records of publication. This term is also appropriately applied to faculty involved primarily in teaching activities as well as to students, especially graduate students, involved in serious investigations on the leading edge of their academic specialties. In liberal learning, basic empiricism in research is not necessarily the standard of faculty productivity. Basic research, often defined by the social and physical sciences as the accumulation of verifiable data, does not rate high within liberal circles. Applied research, investigations with a distinctly practice-oriented outcome, is also given less value because of practical/professional connotations. Rather, liberal-oriented research would focus on theory development and/or verification of existing concepts. Value is placed on thoughtful inquiry into the meaning of relationships and concepts discovered and the development of new conceptualizations and theory building.

This type of scholarship includes work derived from other research, either basic or applied. It might be analysis of research, a synthesis of several lines of investigation, or theory building from existing inquiry. This work might be presented at professional society meetings and conferences. Student learning in this regard would also focus on the generation of new understanding through the intertwining of concepts and relationships discovered in empirical studies into the formulation of theoretical bases for future investigations.

*Service.* Service under the liberal gerontology education alternative represents a far different approach than would service in the professional education sense. Again, in this alternative, concern for theoretical as opposed to practical or scientific advancement precludes the development of knowledge that can be transmitted to the professional practice domain. Service outcomes are likely to be couched in terms of professional association contributions; for instance, the conceptualization of a basic philosophical stance regarding euthanasia is more appropriate than suggestions for the application of scientifically derived medical concepts in professional continuing education. The service orientation of faculty and students most appropriately concentrates on communication with peer groups within the university and with learned societies rather than on consultation with service providers or government agencies.

In general, the liberal gerontology education outcomes suggest that faculty expect for students, and students for themselves, not direct utility of education but the furtherance of learning for its own sake. An instructional program of this type is typically located within a liberal arts or multiversity setting. The costs associated with the educational methodology accompanying this orientation (e.g., small classes, seminars, emphasis on small teacher-student ratio, considerable faculty-student contact, etc.) suggest that only the well endowed, often private liberal arts colleges could develop an accountability system justifying such an expensive program. The high costs of this methodology represent the emphasis on fewer students in ratio to employed faculty, thus reducing the all important credit hour production so necessary for many academic units to survive in this time of limited resources. This alternative would not be practical for community colleges, traditional four-year institutions, or moderate sized universities because the generally held perception is that these institutions support and promote either scientifically oriented training or professional education.

## Pursuing New Knowledge: Scientific Gerontology Education

The second way to arrive at outcomes for gerontology education is to replicate in the study of aging various approaches used by other disciplines. Purposes associated with this scientific gerontology education include content depth and an understanding of gerontology as a distinct field of endeavor. Truth is the goal of this approach and, in this context, is "more related to current facts, including facts about the physical universe, and is always being discovered and tested and applied anew" (Carnegie Commission on Higher Education, 1973, p. 84). Specialized scientific education of this type is characterized by Henderson and Henderson (1975) as employing the concept of "intensive study." They suggest that intellectual training should "concentrate on a problem and a field of knowledge. It should include development of the skills of observation, the collection of information and the testing of validity and reliability, and the carrying through processes to conclusions that are based on skillfully analyzed facts" (p. 100). Scientific gerontology education is likely to be characterized as a narrow, intensive, and unidisciplinary study, one that falls at the opposite end of a continuum from liberal gerontology education.

The instructional program associated with scientific gerontology education of necessity includes a clear sequence of courses oriented toward the development of narrowly defined scientific knowledge. There is a strong emphasis on the fundamentals of the basic disciplines associated with gerontology such as the biology of aging. Students are expected to demonstrate a deep understanding of the scientific principles and methodology associated with a disciplinary endeavor and to be able to identify the unique and specialized applications of these to a discrete aspect of the aging process.

   *Organization of studies.* Outcomes for this type of instructional program would relate to (1) student mastery of discipline-based methodologies, (2) understanding of the principles and knowledge which historically have been generated, and (3) demonstration of skill in recalling the pertinent facts and concepts in selected portions of the field. Limited emphasis is placed on the interdisciplinary implications of the data, with more emphasis on the strictly disciplinary aspects. Students perceive of themselves as becoming scientists in an academic specialty with a concentrated focus on aging.

Faculty members committed to the scientific approach to gerontology education are oriented toward training students in the disciplinary skills of research methodology. There is a heavy reliance on role-modeling, in which the student works closely with a faculty member in the laboratory or on a project that will serve to test the knowledge and skills the student has developed. This apprenticeship approach is often spread over several years at the graduate level and enables the student to gain much practical experience before receiving his "union card" in the form of a research-oriented advanced degree.

*Faculty orientation to the subject matter.* The faculty member is committed to the search for new knowledge in a clearly defined area. Professional advancement results from publication of research and teaching, developing scientists rather than providing service to the local community. Relationships with the national and international scientific community are likely to be more meaningful than local relationships with faculty from other departments in the college or university. Thus, a cosmopolitan outlook is maintained rather than a local orientation. Cosmopolitanism suggests that faculty derive their professional frame of reference from the national or international colleagueship.

*Credentials.* Graduation from a scientific gerontology education program is likely to result in a terminal degree (typically the Ph.D.) and indicates the readiness of the student to accept his/her place within the research and teaching community. Although it does not automatically follow that graduates will seek employment in institutions of higher education, this is a likely outcome and one viewed as appropriate by faculty and graduates. Other possibilities include government or private laboratories, consultant firms, or publishing companies. In each case, the positions will require great technical knowledge and skill.

The baseline undergraduate credential is likely to be the bachelor's degree, usually viewed as a stepping stone to more advanced education: a graduate program in the same discipline (e.g., biology, psychology, or political science) or entry into an associated professional school such as medicine, psychological counseling, or law. The gerontology interest developed at the undergraduate level may well become a primary determinant of the particular graduate school chosen, since not all programs offer gerontology emphases at the professional or doctoral level.

*Research.* Research for the scientific gerontology educator is most closely aligned with narrowly defined, empirical research. Again referring to the Carnegie Commission (1973):

> The purpose of learning is not so much to reinforce or to find the moral precepts and intellectual bulwarks of a more value-oriented society. Rather, it is to devote itself to "the improvement of man's lot" in a society traveling upward, by way of scientific discovery, on the road called Progress [p. 84].

This orientation suggests outcomes of a highly specialized and rigorously defined nature. The knowledge explosion of the 20th century requires that scientific exploration pursue the minute details of the disciplines in order to be classified as a true contribution to the growth of knowledge. Student activities in research focus on documenting previously held knowledge of a small part of a larger whole, and experimental research focuses on the microstructure of a particular aspect of science.

Research outcomes of scientific gerontology are reported in scholarly publications such as the *Journal of Gerontology.* These tend to emphasize the medical and biological aspects of the field. This is not to suggest that the social sciences do not also have a place in scientific gerontology education. However, more time is required before the methodologies and content of gerontology will emerge fully as subspecialties in these "soft sciences."

Many current programs, especially at the graduate level, have begun to make significant strides in furthering the disciplinary base of social gerontology. Student and faculty research are increasingly evident in publications and professional society programs and more data generation seems sure to occur in the future.

*Service.* As with liberal gerontology, scientific gerontology educators are likely to become involved with service activities directly related to the professional and scientific peer group rather than to community service agencies. Many research and teaching outcomes have direct application to service, albeit at a highly specialized level, but such outcomes clearly have secondary priority when compared to scholarly, empirical presentations. The service outcomes are evaluated by their contribution to the furtherance of scientifically based knowledge, the inclusion of that knowledge in teaching, and the generation of new questions for further explication.

One service outcome of scientific gerontology is service of faculty as consultants to laboratories, clinics, and other educational institutions, sharing their findings. Consultation with federal government agencies attempting to solve major social problems might occur if the agency desired to understand more fully the related biological findings. However, this type of application is very limited and leads to the common criticism that service agencies and institutions are unable to integrate highly specific, scientific knowledge into their day-to-day operations.

Scientific gerontology education outcomes must be stringently focused on purposes associated with depth, primacy, and academic rigor. The expectations of faculty for students encompass the mastery of knowledge and methods associated with a primary discipline and the integration of specialized gerontological knowledge into this basic conceptual scheme. This alternative would appear to be inappropriate for location in a community or junior college, a comprehensive four-year college, or a liberal arts institution. Programs employing these outcomes and purposes are highly technical and require a fairly sophisticated graduate school, similar to those usually found in the major national multiversities and selected private universities with specialized faculty, research laboratories, and related resources. The high prestige accorded this type of program requires an outstanding faculty and a history of high program quality and productivity. These prerequisites will limit the number of this type of gerontology education program. However, there appears to be a place for programs that offer master's degrees to form alliances with major institutions in order to develop a curricular hierarchy focusing on the preparation of scientific scholars for gerontology.

## Social Intervention:
## Professional Gerontology Education

The third and final set of alternative outcomes of gerontology education is the most predominant and relevant in the opinion of many gerontology educators. This alternative, professional gerontology education, has as its primary concern the application of knowledge to existing social problems. Professionalism is the usable commodity of higher education; it is viewed as the one output of colleges and universities that can be quantified in terms of direct cost-effectiveness measures in the production of graduates.

A primary general outcome of professional education is what Anderson (1977) describes as "professional identity" (p. 15). The purpose of professional education in gerontology is to produce graduates who look, act, and think like professional gerontologists. The definition of "professional" provided by Schein (1972) allows us to formulate a general understanding of the purposes and ultimate outcomes for gerontology education in the professional vein and to assess whether gerontology can meet these definitional requirements. Schein provides the following points of definition:

1. The professional, as distinct from the amateur, is engaged in a *full-time occupation* that comprises his principal source of income.
2. The professional is assumed to have a *strong motivation* or calling as a basis for his choice of a professional career and is assumed to have a stable lifetime commitment to that career.
3. The professional possesses a *specialized body of knowledge and skills* that are acquired during a *prolonged period of education and training.*
4. The professional makes his decisions on behalf of a client in terms of *general principles, theories, or propositions,* which he applies to the particular case under consideration. . . .
5. At the same time, the professional is assumed to have a *service orientation,* that means that he uses his expertise on behalf of the particular needs of his client.
6. The professional's service to the client is assumed to be based on the *objective needs of the client* and independent of the particular sentiments that the professional may have about the client.
7. The professional is assumed to know better what is good for the client than the client himself. In other words, the professional demands *autonomy of his own performance.*
8. Professionals form *professional associations which define criteria of admission, educational standards, licensing or other formal entry examinations, career lines within the profession, and areas of jurisdiction for the profession.*
9. Professionals have great power and status in the area of their expertise, but their *knowledge is assumed to be specific.* A professional does not have a license to be a "wise man" outside the area defined by his training.
10. Professionals make their service available but ordinarily are *not allowed to advertise or to seek out clients* [pp. 8-9].

Obviously, the professional gerontologist would not have to subject his profession to all the criteria listed by Schein. It would seem appropriate, however, for a would-be professional to meet most of the criteria in order to achieve some minimally established standard for use of the designation. Professional gerontology education, then, seeks to provide an environment and program of studies oriented to the particular trappings of its profession and provides the necessary experiences and role models so that students can achieve "professional identity" as well as professional competence in the field of aging.

*Organization of studies.* Teaching outcomes for professional gerontology education are in most instances founded upon a broadly based understanding of aging. The instruction can be housed either in a primary organizational unit or in an ancillary support unit, but it always focuses on those ideals that relate to some type of professional practice. The ultimate goal is the preparation of students for the work of gerontology. Although gerontology educators have difficulty in providing an operational definition of a "gerontologist," instructional programs are nevertheless endeavoring to provide education toward the end of becoming a professional gerontologist.

Teaching outcomes in professional gerontology education are eminently practical. They relate to the knowledge and skills students will need for successful employment in agencies and institutions providing services to older people. This means that there will be little emphasis on liberal understandings or disciplinary depth. Rather, an appreciation of the client and his needs, wants, and preferences will be combined with knowledge of the various types of intervention and understanding of the current community service system. Specific outcomes include mastery of skills in the areas of human relations, management, program planning, service development, group processes, and evaluation. The application of knowledge is much more important than theoretical reflection and/or scientific investigation.

Faculty members expect students to demonstrate an understanding of the implications of empirically derived knowledge to the particular field of practice. Students in turn expect to be provided with the knowledge and skills necessary to secure and hold positions of increasing responsibility in professional practice. Teaching methods reflect an emphasis on experiential learning, whether in specific courses or as the culminating field practice experience required in most professional programs of study.

*Faculty orientation to subject matter.* Faculty involved in professional education often come to academe from a period of practice in a community agency or institution. This experience generally provides an understanding of the real world of service delivery and the skills students will need in order to survive and prosper in the years ahead. This expertise is manifested in an interest in developing and utilizing specific approaches to needs assessment, intervention, or program development. The design of program plans, community assessment instruments, diagnostic devices, and evaluation measures will be viewed by the student as directly helpful and appropriate to future needs.

Faculty also develop and maintain close professional contacts with the service community. Membership in the local professional associations, community activism, and direct service through private practice or consultation are maintained and encouraged. The content of the field comprises a better understanding of the problems of the client group, of the inadequacies of society generally, and of the means to correct the situation. The orientation is toward service and the client rather than to the academic sphere.

*Credentials.* Completion of a program of professional gerontology education leads to a degree that opens admission to the field of service. In some cases this means licensing or certification as a professional. In gerontology at this time, it means that the individual can present a transcript of course and field work that indicates preparation for human service within an institutional or community setting. The degree typically is not designed to lead to advanced study but is generally considered to be the terminal degree in the field.

Professional gerontology education, then, prepares the individual to enter the field of practice by knowing the current problems of the client group, by understanding the current delivery system of services, and by developing the skills perceived to be necessary in providing service. Although there is currently no universally accepted license, degree, or certificate for this purpose in gerontology, many institutions of higher education are moving in this direction and preparing persons for service roles of this type.

*Research.* Research for faculty and students in the professional gerontology education alternative is most often described as "applied research." For those of the scientific school, this term may be considered pejorative, but many external funding agencies perceive this type of research to hold the highest value for the near-term solution to social problems. Research outcomes typically have direct applicability to the pressing needs of the elderly and are judged on the perceived utility of the findings rather than on contribution to scientific knowledge.

Research outcomes for professional gerontology education are best described as action research. Many times the research includes an intervention as a significant portion of the project. The relative value of the research, then, is measured in the amount and quality of resulting change in the system. Students involved in action research are often encouraged to assess a project's merits in terms of its utility and practicality rather than its methodological purity. This in no way condemns the scientific rigor employed in applied research projects; the desired outcomes for applied research are significantly different from those of scientific research, as is the use made of the knowledge derived.

*Service.* Public service outcomes for the professional gerontology education program are unlike the outcomes of liberal or scientific education. Direct service components of a particular educational program are designed to implement classroom and research learning. Service opportunities for students can result in personally meaningful transfers of classroom knowledge to the "real world," and faculty can practice what they "preach" in order to bridge the gap between the real world and the ivory tower.

Examples of service outcomes for the professional gerontology education program unit are many: Students intern in local, regional, and national agencies and institutions to test out their skills in a practice setting; faculty act as consultants to governmental and private agencies, broadening their view of the problems and applications that will eventually face their students. While service to the professional community is an important component, service to the field of practice is the highest service achievement. A faculty member's worth to a professional school or program is measured not by his/her publications but rather by the extent of professional consultation.

Programs of professional gerontology education are to be found in all types of institutions, private, public, two-year, four-year, and multiversity. Their popularity is best indicated by the numbers of students enrolled and the practical outcomes expected. The preparation for a job in the confusing, problematical, and "dog-eat-dog" world provides students with a tangible reward upon which they can base their motivation and explanation for attending college. Should an operational definition for the practice of gerontology ever be achieved and employers convinced of the need for college-educated practitioners, professional gerontology education will become, to an even greater extent, the principal mode for gerontology education.

## Conclusion

The outcomes of gerontology education may be divided into three distinct categories: liberal, professional, and scientific. Liberal education has great breadth and introduces the student to an understanding of the meaning and importance of the field. Professional education prepares a student for employment in an agency or institution serving older people and is more skill oriented. Scientific education incorporates the search for truth, so expertise in research procedures is primary. Each of these categories of outcomes has major implications for faculty, student expectations, teaching style, research interest, and relationships with the community.

These three general outcomes provide a foundation for examining the field of gerontology education. It is through the use of this conceptualization that the organizational structures, credentials, curriculum, and faculty for the field will be examined. Thus, the outcomes form the foundation on which much of the following material will be based.

## References

Anderson, K.J. In Defense of Departments. In McHenry, D.E. (ed.). *Academic Departments*. San Francisco: Jossey-Bass, 1977.

Brown, D.G. A Scheme for Measuring the Outputs of Higher Education. In Lawrence, B., G. Weathersby, and V.W. Patterson (eds.). *Outputs of Higher Education: Their Identification, Measurement, and Evaluations*. Boulder, Colo.: Western Interstate Commission on Higher Education, 1970, pp. 26–38.

Brubacher, J.S. *On The Philosophy of Higher Education*. San Francisco: Jossey-Bass, 1977.

Carnegie Commission on Higher Education. *The Purposes and the Performance of Higher Education in the United States*. New York: McGraw-Hill, 1973.

Dressel, P.L., and L.B. Mayhew. *Higher Education as a Field of Study*. San Francisco: Jossey-Bass, 1974.

Henderson, A.D., and J.G. Henderson. *Higher Education in America*. San Francisco: Jossey-Bass, 1975.

Micek, S.S., A.L. Service, and Y.S. Lee. *Outcome Measures and Procedures Manual* (Field Review Edition). Technical Report No. 70. Boulder, Colo.: National Center for Higher Education Management Systems, Western Interstate Commission on Higher Education, May, 1975.

Richman, B.M., and R.N. Farmer. *Leadership, Goals, and Power in Higher Education*. San Francisco: Jossey-Bass, 1974.

Schein, E.H. *Professional Education*. New York: McGraw-Hill, 1972.

# 6

# Administrative Structures for Gerontology Education

Gerontology education within American colleges and universities currently exhibits a wide array of administrative structures. This diversity has resulted from the differing missions and objectives of the educational institutions and the variety of gerontology activity. Some programs had their genesis in the research interests of one or two faculty members and incorporated this investigatory focus into subsequent educational activity. Others emanated from undergraduate instruction, expanded to include courses on the processes of aging. A third category of programs developed in response to the financial incentives offered by government agencies for the preparation of manpower for community and institutional services. The varying beginnings resulted in administrative organizational structures with few similarities.

The organizational structures developed do not automatically fall into any clear or discernible patterns. Many have been modeled after other units within a particular institution, and some have been created as unique entities designed to serve the needs of a program in a new field. In order to begin the process of describing and analyzing these organizational designs, it is first necessary to review briefly some of the literature on administrative structures in higher education. The remainder of the chapter will describe five types of organizational structures that have evolved during the short history of gerontology education.

## Understanding Organizational Structures

Organizational structures in colleges and universities are complex; they vary in level, size, purpose, and operation. This complexity has produced something of a mystique regarding the secrets of organization and administration within institutions of higher learning. While the situation is confusing, there is little if any mystique involved. The determination of organizational structures at both the institutional level and at the primary unit level is based upon several factors. Principal among these is the enabling legislation or charter upon which an institution is based. This documented foundation in most cases describes the mission and intent of the institution of higher education and provides the basis for development of organizational structures. The early Colonial colleges, for example, had a primary mission of cultivating a learned ministry for the settled areas and the frontier. This mission caused the development of departments of religion and, to some extent, the arts. As often as not, there was a great degree of continuity throughout the institution, which was reflected by a highly structured curriculum and by faculty organization. This structure was typical of the liberal arts colleges and continued to be the dominant model into the early 1940s (Rudolph, 1962).

The concept of university organization, as opposed to the earliest colleges, was brought to this country from Germany in the late 1860s. Johns Hopkins University, based upon the German model of the research-focused university, brought about a revolution in the manner in which the work of higher education was undertaken. The principal emphases of the German model as compared to the English college model were deemphasis of students' moral development and a total absorption with students' intellectual development. Faculty no longer were forced to assume custodial roles with students, departments became the enclave for faculty retreat from excessive student interaction, and the laboratory became the principal arena for teaching. The most significant difference between the Colonial college and the research-focused university of that time was a shift in emphasis from student personal development to emphasis on student/faculty intellectual development.

As the German model spread and matured in this country, there finally evolved the concept of university in the true American sense. The University of Virginia established a blending of the research and personal development emphases. This blending of intended educational outcomes is the foundation for many different organizational structures. The proliferation of institutions as civilization advanced across the United States produced the mélange of organizational structures represented in the nation's colleges and universities today.

Some attempts have been made to compare the organization of colleges and universities to other forms of public and private enterprise. Perkins et al. (1973) provide a brief comparison of higher education organization with corporations, government bureaus, large foundations, and other types of institutions. Their general conclusion was that educational institutions are a unique class of organization, comparable to no other in industry or government. Our best approach to the analysis of organizational structures in higher education is to consider the subclasses of structures employed in colleges and universities which constitute the differences among institutions.

Peter Blau (1973) presented a very complicated analysis of quantitative data on 115 American colleges and universities in which the effect of administrative structures on scholarship was discussed. While certainly a scholarly contribution to the study of this complex topic, Blau's premise was that the college or university is in fact a bureaucratic organization. This assumption is disputed by Millett (1962) and Ikenberry (1972); consequently, Blau's conclusions must be viewed as tentative at best.

Moran (1968) suggested that two "interesting and conflicting" organizational models have emerged, "neither supported by research findings but attracting attention nevertheless by reason of the experience and stature of the authors and the insight and logic of their respective presentations" (p. 146). The first model described by Moran is, in his words, "espoused by Millett" and suggests that the organizational basis of American colleges and universities is a community of power rather than the hierarchy of power that exists in a bureaucratic environment. For example, the processes employed in the development and approval of curricula in a collegial department involve a high degree of informal influence and practically no "line authority" decisions. In the truly collegial department, the faculty are more or less a body of equals, attempting to generate decisions and procedures based on consensus, rather than on the authority that one's place within the hierarchy demands. When this concept is utilized in a large university employing hundreds of faculty members, the community-of-power concept suggests that faculty would identify with their colleagues as an institutional grouping rather than accepting any superficial administrative network established to facilitate the housekeeping activities of administrators. Moran also suggests that this position is favored by such noted authorities as Beardsley Ruml and Donald Morrison.

The other model described in Moran's work is promoted by Clark Kerr and Edward Litchfield. In this view, the university is presented as an "organic community with schools and colleges bound to one another by a common goal or goals" (p. 146). This position suggests that the administrative framework ignored in the preceding model would define the interior limits of the organizational structures by which the institution would govern itself. The units associated with a model of this type would tend to be more bureaucratic in nature, more problem centered in focus, and more hiearchical in decision-making processes. This approach to organization would more fittingly be subtitled the "administrators" model as opposed to a community-focused "faculty" model. These dichotomous models provide a potential framework for assessing the organizational structures of a majority of primary academic units involved in gerontology education.

## Organizational Models

The department is the traditional academic unit within colleges and universities; it is the organizational entity that most clearly reflects the concept of a community of power. In most institutions, the department is the smallest unit of organization and provides the faculty with their appointments and institutional identity. The curriculum is developed and offered through departments, which, for most institutions, are the only units authorized to award academic credit. Departmental chairpersons are the primary level administrators within higher education; they are typically representatives of the democratically determined viewpoint and philosophy of the departmental faculty and therefore exemplify the focus of the community of power described by Moran.

Departments have traditionally represented the logical division of the principal disciplines and dominant fields within institutions of higher education. By having a department established, a particular discipline or field creates a structure with the highest degree of refinement achievable within the college or university. This division of knowledge into miniscule departments has often been criticized as inhibiting the development of new conceptualizations, isolating professors, and producing narrowness in curricula and research (Anderson, 1977). On the positive side, departments historically have provided a simple and durable unit that represents the most logical implementation of a community-of-power concept, the traditional intent of collegial organizational philosophy.

The second organizational model described by Moran provides the opportunity for program developers to generate an administrative milieu that moves beyond the traditional concept of academic departments. Ikenberry (1972) describes this model as consisting of task-oriented organizational units, more specific and restricted in mission. Rather than being based upon a disciplinary or content specialization, task-oriented units are typically problem oriented with faculty from several disciplines cooperatively undertaking research, instruction, or community service designed to better understand or eliminate the vicissitudes of a general or specific problem. Often, part-time and jointly appointed faculty participate in the various projects; and involvement may increase or terminate depending upon the current undertakings of the unit.

Ikenberry lists five advantages of task-oriented units. First, by defining a task, the unit will have a more clearly delineated mission, facilitating the formulation of precise statements of function. Second, task orientation encourages the reduction of controls and restrictions placed on traditional departments by the parent institution since the task unit will typically not have the same authority in terms of curricula and faculty. This allows for increased decentralization, which may reduce the dependence on other college or university units. For instance, if the preparation of social workers was the task of a School of Social Work, all requirements and electives could be the prerogative of the school rather than the institution at large.

A third advantage of task-oriented units is their ability to respond positively to new opportunities, consequently increasing the diversity of college and university programs. While departmental structures are criticized for inhibiting the formation of new fields of study (e.g., gerontology), task-oriented units foster interdisciplinary and problem-centered approaches. The fourth advantage is that task-oriented units provide faculty with increased operating autonomy. The less-restricted mission of the unit allows for more involvement in nontraditional instruction, a variety of community undertakings, expanded applied research, and ability to respond quickly to federal grant opportunities. The final advantage is that task-oriented units enhance the institution's control and accountability in carrying out specified missions and tasks. With a precise mission it is possible to clearly describe and control the activities and re-

sources of the unit. Although the development of task-oriented units
has met with some opposition from those whose academic preparation and loyalty are with traditional disciplinary and departmental
structures, task- or problem-centered units have found considerable
use in the field of gerontology.

## Structures for Gerontology Education

The examination of organizational structures in gerontology education may be facilitated by suggesting that existing units fall along a
bimodal continuum. The continuum indicates the extent to which a
particular type of organizational structure is based upon a community-of-power concept or upon a task-oriented concept. Thus on one
end of the continuum are the traditionally organized departments
and at the other end are the task-oriented units, usually identified as
institutes or centers. In employing this continuum for analysis, we
have a basis for distinguishing among the various structures and for
classifying them in relation to the concepts of community of power
and task orientation.

To provide maximum clarity in the following discussion, it has
been necessary to generate five eclectic models of organizational
structure in gerontology education. These descriptive models are
presented as a reasonably comprehensive overview of current gerontology in higher education. Although not every program will fit into
one of these five models, they appear to reflect structures viewed as
the most appropriate, or the most politically advantageous, by institutions at the present time. Neither of the two analyzing concepts—
community of power and task orientation—is totally applicable in
every case. A compromise approach must be used in which the analysis and description of any particular organizational structure will
include the interaction of the concepts rather than the application
of one or the other.

The data from which these five models are derived were gath-
ered in a study of gerontology in higher education by the authors
during 1976-77. This study, supported through a grant from the
✳ Administration on Aging, USDHEW, generated a national data base
on the current state of gerontology instruction in all types of post-
secondary institutions. A major part of this study was an in-depth site
visit and interview of faculty and administrators of 17 institutions
with gerontology education programs. The data and insights from
these interviews, combined with questionnaire responses from 169

institutions, identified the factors effecting initiation and evolution of different types of organizational structures in a variety of institutions (Bolton, 1978). The factors identified were (1) curricula: the courses selected for inclusion in the program of studies; (2) faculty: their appointment status and academic preparation; (3) administration: the nature of communication channels established within and outside of the institution; and (4) students: their intents and the educational outcomes predicted for them. By describing the characteristics and interactions of these factors in a variety of gerontology education program units, it is possible to suggest that five organizational models exist: (1) intradepartmental structures; (2) departments of gerontology; (3) schools of gerontology; (4) interdepartmental committees; and (5) institutes or centers of gerontology. The models represent positions along the continuum with the first, intradepartmental structures, falling near the community-of-power end and the last, institutes, being placed close to the task-oriented end.

*5 models*

## Intradepartmental Structure

The first structural arrangement for gerontology education is an intradepartmental setting, one in which all course offerings are concentrated within one of the established departments of the institution. Typically, the departments that have become hosts for gerontology are psychology, sociology, social work, public administration, nursing, adult education, or a similar discipline or professional field with a strong affinity to gerontology. The determination of which department would provide the most congenial home for gerontology instruction depends upon faculty interest and administrator receptivity. The location often develops from a specific faculty member's interest in gerontology as an adjunct to his/her principal discipline. Thus, the placement evolves through faculty activity and administrative support rather than through any conscious plan.

The curriculum in this model emphasizes those aspects of gerontology which relate most closely to the host discipline or field of study. Thus, a gerontology program within a department of psychology would be likely to include courses on personality aspects of later life, cognitive developments in aging, perception and old age, and clinical applications to the older adult. These courses clearly apply to the field of gerontology, but they do not provide a very broad exposure. They would be likely to ignore totally the social, economic, political, and even the biological aspects of aging. Although the number of available courses would vary from one institution to another, it would be expected that a minimum of two courses would have primarily gerontological content in order for the unit to claim that it had a subunit or intradepartmental gerontology education program (Bolton, 1978).

The instructors responsible for teaching gerontology courses in this model are usually the regular departmental faculty. Although some of them might have academic or experiential preparation in aging, the primary requisite for an appointment in the department is education and/or competence in the discipline or field rather than in gerontology *per se*. As faculty of the department, they would gain their status and rewards by meeting the expectations of the department. Therefore, if the psychology program mentioned above emphasized publication, the faculty member may need to publish in psychology journals as well as to become visible in the gerontology network.

Administration of gerontology instruction occurs through the established departmental channels with the chairperson and the faculty committees having the final responsibility for curriculum, student selection, and faculty assignments. As an intradepartmental activity, gerontology is perceived as an adjunct to the department's program of studies and does not require independent academic administration.

Students enrolled in the gerontology curriculum would first be students of the principal department and only secondarily be involved in the study of gerontology. Their admission, counseling, and graduation would be guided and administered by the department. In this manner, the study of gerontology is a part of and completely subject to the authority and regulation of the host department. There is little or no opportunity for faculty members or students to develop gerontology programs, since gerontology is an adjunct rather than an organizational entity.

The intradepartmental structure provides the least autonomy of the five models to be cited. The concept of "community of power" has limited usefulness here since the number of faculty and the viability of their influence would be quite restricted. The faculty of the department have most of the power, and although they operate within the guidelines of the community-power principle, the gerontology faculty are clearly minority partners. There is the potential for the gerontology faculty to have some independent identity and influence. This is not likely to occur in most cases because the host department will maintain its emphasis on the discipline or field of study and will restrict gerontology's growth if it threatens to become too strong.

The intradepartmental model has one significant advantage to recommend it: An institution with limited resources can initiate a series of courses in gerontology without committing the funding necessary to establish an independent academic unit. However, this situation may prove to be a disadvantage at some point in the growth process. Because there is no commitment to institutionalize the program, it may never achieve the permanence desired. Thus, the two major drawbacks of this model are that students are able to gain an understanding of only a limited aspect of gerontology and that the program is likely to remain dependent upon the personal interest of one or two faculty members without substantial institutional support. For those institutions unwilling or unable to devote significant resources to the establishment of an independent program in gerontology, this type of organizational arrangement allows an acceptable alternative which may provide the basis for establishment of a more comprehensive program in the future.

## A Department of Gerontology

The second organizational model, a department of gerontology, closely resembles the community of power described by Moran. By virtue of its designation, the department of gerontology would have the authority and prerogative afforded all departments within the institution. The exact meaning of the concept community of power would be determined by the traditional place and status given departments in the institution. For the most part, department chairpersons are accorded positions of considerable stature in traditional and mature institutions. Their representation of the faculty within the administration hierarchy provides a strong position in relation to other administrators and upholds the traditional values of collegial governance.

The curriculum of a gerontology department includes a series of courses that can be selected as a major or minor for traditional degrees. In some cases, a professional degree such as the Master of Science in Gerontology is offered. The courses would be listed under the designations associated with the department and credit-hour production would be assigned to the department in the typical manner. In some instances, gerontology courses may be offered by cooperating departments; however, these courses would not carry a primary gerontology designation. Cross-listing of such courses between departments would be a common occurrence in many institutions. The curriculum would include gerontology courses taught from several perspectives. Students would be able to gain an understanding of the social, psychological, and physical aspects of aging as well as exposure to economic, political, and human service elements of the field.

In this model, the gerontology faculty would have the gerontology department as their primary (or exclusive) source of academic appointment. Decisions regarding rank, promotion, and tenure would be made by the department, with other units having some limited involvement in the case of joint appointees. Although some departments would have nonteaching staff involved primarily in research or community service, this would be less likely than in more task-oriented units. Faculty status and rewards would be closely tied to the mission of the gerontology department. If publications were emphasized, articles appearing in gerontological journals would be the most highly regarded, and formal preparation in gerontological research would be desired.

A gerontology department would evidence an administrative structure similar to that of the traditional departments within the particular institution. It is important to note that there exists a high degree of variability among institutions regarding the independence and collegial governance which departments are allowed. In this discussion, the ideal of collegiality is assumed. A chairperson would be more common than a director or similarly titled administrator. A variety of faculty committees would lessen the bureaucratic nature of the organization by allowing decision making to be located within the community of power rather than within a hierarchical structure.

As a traditional department, gerontology would, of necessity, be a part of a larger administrative body such as a college or division. There are numerous alternatives for placement within the institution, and no standard locus has been determined. Colleges or divisions having a public service, community service, or human services emphasis are quite often selected for professionally oriented units, but academic or scientific units may be located in a variety of settings.

In a gerontology department, students would be admitted, counseled, instructed, and supervised by the gerontology faculty. No admission to other academic units would be necessary, and no unit would be likely to have any specific influence over giving credits. External controls placed on student courses would include institutional regulations and requirements regarding specific forms of degrees (e.g., the differences that might exist in the awarding of a B.S. as opposed to a B.A.)

The department of gerontology has many advantages over the intradepartmental structure. For those concerned with institutional legitimacy and survival, and their numbers are growing each year, the department offers the most secure organizational structure. The department, in practically all institutions, is allocated "hard money lines", which become a permanent part of the institutional budget (to the extent any budget line is permanent in these times of budget cuts and retrenchment). On the other hand, the creation of a departmental structure is difficult since the requirements and procedures for establishment are often quite rigorous. In some cases, a new department is viewed by existing units as an invasion of their territory and vigorously opposed. The competition for scarce resources makes many, if not most, institutions extremely hesitant about allowing the formation of a new department while program reductions may be occurring elsewhere in the institution. This process, however, seldom occurs while a given unit retains any life. Therefore, departments have many attractive features for program developers, but institutional realities may preclude this organizational structure in many institutions.

## A School of Gerontology

A school of gerontology would represent a position on the continuum somewhere near the midpoint between departmental structures and task-oriented units. The nature of professional schools in most universities suggests a mode of operation more autonomous than a department but displaying less independence than a center or institute. As a semi-independent affiliate of a university, the school would recruit and select its own students, employ its own faculty, offer majors and/or degrees, and have its own administrative structure equivalent to other professional schools within the institution. This model suggests that gerontology would be viewed as a separate discipline or, more appropriately in the case of professional schools, as a professional field of endeavor.

For the school of gerontology, the curriculum would likely be well developed and provide access to many facets of the field from both theoretical and practical viewpoints. Rather than having other departments or academic units offer gerontology instruction in a cooperative multidisciplinary fashion, the school of gerontology would employ faculty with broad and diverse academic backgrounds in order to offer a full range of gerontology instruction. Usually, the curriculum would deemphasize scholarly rigor and would stress the knowledge and skills needed for successful professional practice. This type of curriculum suggests that specialization is important only to the extent that it relates to specified educational outcomes, and for the majority of schools, this outcome is professional competence.

The faculty of a school of gerontology would have their primary appointments in the school. Because few faculty members currently hold a doctorate in gerontology, joint appointments with other departments may be sought by some who desire to maintain identification with their discipline or field of origin. Decisions on appointment, promotion, and tenure would obviously be the prerogative of the school. Emphasis would likely be placed on gerontology research, publication, and service rather than on activities in the field of origin.

Administratively, a school of gerontology would be headed by a director or dean, assisted by various faculty committees. Within the parameters set by the parent institution, the school would govern itself as an independent academic unit. The location of a school of gerontology within the college or university structure would depend upon whether the school was considered to be a semiautonomous academic unit similar to a college of the university or was parallel to a traditional department and therefore placed within a particular college. If it were a semiautonomous unit, the dean or director would report to the principal academic officer and the unit would be equal to other colleges. In the latter case, however, placement within the institution would be of concern. The typical location of professional gerontology education programs would be with other human service units in a college of community service or public affairs. The placement of a professional school within a college structure is unlikely; typically, professional education units have the functions and authority of a college.

Student recruitment, counseling, instruction, and recommendation for degrees would be within the authority of the school. The students would take the bulk of their instruction from school faculty with a minimum of outside electives being allowed. The emphasis would be placed on the socialization process necessary to become a practicing gerontologist. Field experience, professionally oriented courses, and awareness of the contemporary condition of older people would be paramount. The students would concentrate their attention on gerontology rather than concerning themselves with liberal or broadening study.

While a higher degree of autonomy and internal control is part of the attractiveness of a school of gerontology, there are limited examples of this type of structure currently in operation. The resources necessary for the establishment of a school are great enough to preclude most institutions from considering this alternative. The only existing school of gerontology in this country was established with an endowment of significant proportions. This fortunate occurrence is rare; therefore this alternative, no matter how desireable, is unlikely to be feasible to any but the best-endowed institutions.

## An Interdepartmental Committee on Gerontology

An interdepartmental committee on gerontology offers the opportunity for cooperation among several departments in the development of inter- or multidisciplinary educational experiences in gerontology. It would be placed on the task-oriented end of the continuum and would exhibit a high degree of autonomy, limited only by the goals and mission of the institution within which it existed. This model represents the first variation of Moran's concept of the organic community approach to organizational structures. Its autonomy and interdepartmental nature would remove it from any established and recognized community of power. Therefore, within the established goals of the institution, an interdepartmental committee would act as an autonomous body without the traditional constraints of organizational structure and lines of communication.

The curriculum of an interdepartmental committee would be composed of a combination of new or existing courses coordinated to provide a comprehensive view of the field of aging. Since gerontology does not reside within any single discipline or field, courses from several different departments would be organized into a planned program of study. The interdepartmental curriculum would offer a concentration in aging associated with traditional degrees or, in some instances, an interdisciplinary degree or credential in gerontology.

Faculty involved in an interdepartmental committee would be members of one or another of the academic departments, divisions, or professional schools of the institution. They would retain their primary assignment with that unit, be governed by the policies of that unit, and be associated with the interdepartmental committee as a supplement to their major assignment. The faculty would join together, however, to form an ad hoc committee that collectively would determine a course sequence and/or approve courses for inclusion in the gerontology concentration or degree. These same faculty would teach the gerontology courses, which might be offered exclusively by the departments or might be cross-listed with the interdepartmental committee so that they could carry a gerontology prefix.

Administrative organization for this model is minimal. A secretary or administrative assistant or, in larger programs, a full-time faculty/administrator would facilitate the functioning of the committee. Outside grants or contracts awarded to the committee would possibly enlarge the number of personnel involved in committee activities, but appointments would usually be temporary in nature and not tenure eligible. The location of an interdepartmental committee within the organization of an institution presents a more complex problem than in the cases of intradepartmental, departmental, or school models. Since degrees may be offered, accountability must reside with some degree- and/or credit-granting unit within the college or university. For this reason, either the interdepartmental committee would be housed within an existing college, school, or division, or the committee would report to the principal academic officer of the institution (a vice-president of academic affairs, dean of the college, etc.). The placement of the committee under the administrative umbrella of the chief academic administrator is the most plausible arrangement since the committee would have the benefit of serving the needs and aspirations of the entire institution rather than only a select department or college. Turf issues are also lessened when the committee is allowed college- or university-wide status.

Authority for the admission of students to an interdepartmental committee program would lie with the committee. It would have the power to admit, advise, and recommend concentrations or degrees, whichever were offered. In many cases, the committee administers only a concentration and any decision on admission, advisement, and award of a degree is the prerogative and responsibility of the department. In the case of interdisciplinary degree programs in gerontology, a faculty member of the committee would assume the responsibility for advising and guiding the program of studies as prescribed by the interdepartmental committee.

Overall, then, the interdepartmental committee model offers a more organizationally decentralized administrative structure for the functions of admissions, program requirements, curriculum, and program development in gerontology. The advantage of this organizational model is that, as with an intradepartmental model, institutional resources are primarily committed to programs of the principal departments. However, a variety of courses and even a degree in gerontology can be initiated without having to establish an independent administrative unit for that purpose. The interdepartmental committee does not typically allow, however, for the institutionalization of gerontology instruction as an independent organizational entity. This may prove to be a major drawback in times of declining resources since the designation of a separate structural entity—a department—may indicate a real commitment to permanence.

## A Center or Institute of Gerontology

The final model of organizational structure represents the furthest movement toward the task-oriented end of the continuum. An institute or center provides the highest level of autonomy while also facilitating interdepartmental cooperation within the goals of the institution. The institute or center is a very sophisticated form of task-oriented academic unit with high levels of the membership in an organic community, as discussed by Moran.

The gerontology curriculum in centers or institutes would be comprised of courses offered by several departments within the institution. Although the center or institute typically cannot teach credit courses as an independent academic unit, it does have the ability to exercise some control over the courses by offering a certificate or other type of credential to students who complete a prescribed course of study. Thus, the courses developed and offered by academic departments become the curriculum for a recognized credential awarded by the institute or center. Often, affiliated departments will consider a specialization or concentration as a minor in conjunction with the degree programs they offer, but this is typically an individually negotiated arrangement between the center or institute and each degree-granting department. The curriculum for these credential programs would be directed by the center or institute through encouraging the affiliated departments to offer "approved" courses. This approval mechanism may then generate additional enrollments in a particular department, a result that becomes more popular as student credit hour production is encouraged in departmental accountability decisions.

Faculty involved in gerontology instruction in this model would not usually hold appointments solely with the center or institute. Rather, their primary appointment would be in the academic departments, and occasionally they would hold adjunct appointments as members of the center or institute staff. Funding for faculty appointments would typically fall to the principal departments; the assignment of specific courses and final decisions on appointment, promotion, and tenure would be the responsibility of the department.

The administrative arrangement for this model tends to be autonomous and task oriented. Typically, center and institute staff engage in a variety of activities in addition to possible teaching assignments. These activities include administration of continuing education for professionals; public information regarding the activities of the center or institute; educational materials and curriculum development; applied and basic research; technical assistance to agencies and institutions; maintenance of specialized library resources; and provision of some direct services as related to the role of the educational institution.

Centers and institutes exist outside the traditional departmental structure of the institution. The unit would be most advantageously placed under the authority of the chief academic officer. In a few instances, centers or institutes might be located within a college or division encompassing a grouping of community, public, or human service fields. This location, however, does not afford the degree of autonomy and institution-wide purview needed for optimal functioning, nor does it allow for the operation of the completely task-oriented mission characteristic of this model.

Students involved in the instructional or credential programs of a center or institute would be admitted to two different but complementary programs. Admission to a degree-granting department would be necessary for pursuit of a traditional degree, and admission to the credential program administered by the institute or center would be required for completion of a specialization or concentration in aging. Thus, a dual system of admissions and program planning should be provided for students pursuing a traditional degree with a credential in gerontology if they wish to be awarded both simultaneously.

Organizational structures in gerontology education represented by this model are becoming quite popular alternatives for many institutions today. Congressional appropriations for Title IV-C, "Multidisciplinary Centers of Gerontology," have promoted this model and provided funding for the development and operation of centers in 43 colleges and universities. For many institutions this structural model represents the most efficient and viable organization; it has proven to be both effective and feasible in many settings. For some institutions, however, the establishment of a center or institute represents an ungainly attempt at replicating the arrangements employed by some of the most notable programs in the country, a replication that is impossible because institutional mission, goals, functions, or administrative schema will not accommodate this design. Intrainstitutional politics and traditions may preclude this alternative for many colleges and universities, and its adoption should be undertaken only after a thorough assessment of the purposes and structures of the parent institution has been made.

## The Issue of Organizational Placement

Where a gerontology education program will be placed within the administrative framework of an institution is crucial. This decision should be made after consideration of several key issues: (1) the traditional organization of the institution; (2) the orientation of primary faculty and administrators involved in the planned program; (3) the current and potential resources available for the establishment, development, and continuation of a program of gerontology studies; and (4) the primary goals and intents of the proposed program.

Tradition within a given institution will dictate the possible alternative structures for emerging programs in gerontology. If an institution has established precedents regarding the nature of credit-awarding units and this tradition excludes one or more of the aforementioned models, the viable alternatives will be limited. Colleges organized around departmental units which have not previously considered the use of interdepartmental committees, institutes, or centers will require extensive efforts to establish these structural models. Multiversities exhibit a wide range of organizational forms and, therefore, provide few obstacles to the development of task-oriented units within the existing framework.

The organizational placement of gerontology education within the college or university often is determined by the location of the interested faculty. Many programs have developed because a faculty member had a persistent interest in gerontology as it relates to his/her principal discipline or field and promoted the establishment of an independent or quasi-autonomous program of studies in aging. Frequently a grant or contract is secured for gerontological education, thus locating the program of studies within or in relation to that faculty member's home department or unit. Through this process gerontology education units have been established in practically every conceivable academic and/or administrative unit within institutions of higher education. Placement of a program based upon the interests of certain faculty, however, does not necessarily represent the most appropriate nor the most effective model. Very often programs established in this manner and funded by "soft money" have a limited life span or are severely restricted in scope. Faculty groups representing the interests of several different academic areas have been more successful in establishing interdepartmental committees or free-standing departments of gerontology, structures expected to experience greater stability (Bolton, 1978).

Financial resources play an important role in determining the placement of gerontology instructional programs. Grants initiated by the central academic administration of an institution typically result in the development of interdepartmental committees, institutes, centers, or quasi-interdisciplinary programs, placed in the central administrative structure. If a given department or academic unit secures monies for the establishment of gerontology instruction, the program will likely become a subunit of that department or will be closely associated with the academic entity that secured the funding.

Ideally, the purposes, goals, and intended educational outcomes would be the appropriate basis for determining the placement of gerontology education within an institution of higher learning. Through the examination of goals and purposes, the program could be placed with other programs espousing the same ideals. Therefore, if the primary goal and purpose of a given program were to prepare health professionals for long-term care settings, the program of studies would ideally be placed with other academic programs oriented toward professional health care education rather than in the college of arts and sciences. One could speculate that the high degree of change in the placement and structure of gerontology education today is a direct result of programs having previously been placed according to the first three methods rather than decisions being made on the basis of program goals and purposes.

## Implications and Trends

These five organizational models for gerontology education do not exhaust the possibilities for instructional arrangements available for programs developers. Some structures are likely to combine elements of several of the models, while others may be totally different from any of the five suggested. For instance, in some colleges and universities the instructional thrust is toward experiential education with field practica and noncredit seminars designed to heighten the student's interests in the field of aging. These programs often have a tenuous structure, depending primarily upon a few faculty members who have personal interest and commitment to the field.

Perhaps more useful than any assessment of the definitive nature of the suggested models are the implications that may be drawn from them. The organizational structures for gerontology education are primarily an indication of the extent of control the faculty exert in the formulation of an instructional program. The departmental model end of the continuum, which employs the community of power concept, represents faculty control and authority over curricula, program requirements, and student admissions. The middle ground on our continuum indicates an attempt to effect an amalgam of both faculty control and task orientations. The interdisciplinary, task-oriented models are more goal directed and thus require greater administrative control over a dispersed and diverse faculty. Some gerontology educators assert that only by exercising careful control over the development and operation of gerontology instruction can the curriculum be directed precisely enough to allow graduates the necessary interdisciplinary depth and skills essential for a sound education and marketable employment skills. With control vested in several academic units, for example, the outcome for students could be neither good sociology nor good gerontology.

Gerontology education structures are in a state of flux. Little consistency is evident since programs vary with institutional requirements, faculty initiation, funding genesis, and recency of development. This time of confusion may be the prelude to a shaking out of the weaker or more inappropriate units, but it appears that it will be some time until there is a typical or modal gerontology education structure.

## References

Anderson, K. J. In Defense of Departments. In McHenry, D. E., et al. (eds.). *Academic Departments.* San Francisco: Jossey-Bass, 1977.

Blau, P. M. *The Organization of Academic Work.* New York: John Wiley and Sons, 1973.

Bolton, C. R. *Gerontology Education in the United States.* Omaha, Neb.: University of Nebraska, 1978.

Ikenberry, S. O. The Organizational Dilemma. *Journal of Higher Education,* 1972, *43,* 23–34.

Millett, J. D. *The Academic Community.* New York: McGraw-Hill, 1962.

Moran, W. E. The Study of University Organizations. *Journal of Higher Education*, 1968, *39*, 144–151.

Perkins, J. A. (ed.). *The University as an Organization*. New York: McGraw-Hill, 1973.

Rudolph, F. *The American College and University*. New York: Random House, 1962.

# 7

# Credentials in Gerontology Education

The awarding of credentials in higher education is a practice first begun in the 12th century. It has progressed dramatically from the simple conferring of the Bachelor's, Master's, and Doctor's degrees to a complex system of degrees and certificates representing a variety of outcomes for higher education instruction.

In the earliest universities, giving credentials filled the dual purpose of signifying the completion of the bachelor of arts and certifying faculty as competent for teaching in the medieval university. The designations of degrees so familiar to present-day educators were not nearly so easily differentiated in the early Middle Ages. The "masters," those certified to teach in the universities, were distinguished from others who had completed the "bachelor of arts" by their admission to the guild of scholars. These early credentials comprised the license to teach and were a requirement for entry into the guild of masters (Stewart, 1967).

Awarding credentials in American higher education was originally built upon the venerable foundation of English and European institutions. Early American colleges typically awarded only one degree, the Bachelor of Arts. This credential represented a broad-based liberal arts education with heavy emphasis on moral instruction and preparation for the clergy or general public service (Rudolph, 1962). With the development of American institutions of graduate education came the proliferation of degrees.

Until the time of the awarding of the first earned Master of Arts, *pro meritis,* the master's degree was often considered an honorary award for those with a bachelor's degree who performed some further work of scholarship or service. With the establishment of the earned Master of Arts at the University of Michigan in 1853 and the offering of an earned Doctor of Philosophy by Yale in 1860, graduate education was formalized in the United States. By the end of the 19th century, the number of degree alternatives began to expand rapidly, until, by 1960, some 2,400 different degree types were awarded in the United States (Spurr, 1970). The problem of understanding the variety and number of degrees available today resembles the selection of automobile models: For all the names and model variations, beneath the surface most are unexcitingly similar with interchangeable components and only superficial, cosmetic differences.

## Degree Structures

There are five levels of degree structures in American higher educational institutions today. These degree levels represent the hierarchy of academic achievement specified for a variety of institutions. The degree levels are arranged and evaluated in terms of the amount of time (number of years) spent in achieving a given level. In most instances satisfactory completion of one level will allow entry into the successive level. There are, however, some exceptions to this pattern. For example, the Master's degree is not a prerequisite for many Ph.D. or professional doctoral programs. Neither is the Specialist in Education a prerequisite for the doctorate in the field of education. There are, however, some logically successive steps in the degree structure and some general frameworks available to help in understanding the various levels within the overall structure.

*Certificates and diplomas.* Not included in the degree hierarchy are several credential alternatives to degrees that have developed over the years. At all levels of higher education—community or junior college, college, and university—credentials are available that represent the completion of a coordinated and supervised program of educational activity that does not fit with traditional degree requirements. Certificates and diplomas represent the successful completion of short courses, whether for college credit or for other forms of credit (e.g., continuing education). These credentials are available at the community or junior college level for the completion of vocational courses that are shorter than the typical two-year associate's degree. Many community or junior college certificate and diploma programs represent courses of study for paraprofessional roles such as nurses' aides, specialized mechanics occupations, or food handling positions.

Programs offered by colleges and universities at the undergraduate level which culminate in the awarding of certificates or diplomas are numerous. The certificate is probably the most common credential at the undergraduate level while the diploma represents intermediate levels of graduate education. Certificates are less likely to be available for work beyond the baccalaureate, as graduate programs tend to involve highly concentrated periods of study not easily adapted to reduced time frames and shortened curricula. The diploma programs intermediate between the master's and doctor's degrees offer a credential especially popular in colleges of education (often referred to as Educational Specialists). Some certificates of specialization are available for graduate level work; however, these concentrated programs are more likely to be noted on student records as minors or cognates rather than being formalized by a separate credential.

### Associate's Degrees

There are essentially two types of associate's degrees that warrant consideration in a discussion of gerontology education: the terminal associate's degree and the transfer associate's degree. In the first instance, the terminal nature of the degree suggests that the curriculum is not appropriate for application toward the completion of the next level, the Bachelor's degree. Terminal associate's degrees are quite often designated as "Associate of Science" or "Associate of Applied Science in Geriatrics." These degrees indicate the completion of a coordinated two-year program of studies in preparation for an applied or paraprofessional occupation. The traditional college courses offered at the freshman and sophomore level are often not included in a terminal associate's degree unless, in the case of written and verbal communication, they are perceived as essential tools for persons functioning at a more sophisticated level.

The transfer associate's degree, often designated an Associate of Arts, represents a traditional freshman and sophomore course of study of general education appropriate for most bachelor's degree programs. The purpose of the transfer degree is twofold: the recipient may in fact choose to transfer as a junior to a baccalaureate degree granting institution,or, on the other hand, the recipient may choose to terminate his/her academic career upon the completion of two years of general education beyond high school. In any case, the associate's degree, typically awarded by community or junior colleges, is the first level of the American hierarchy of degree structures.

## Bachelor's Degrees

Defining and describing the multiple variations of the baccalaureate is no simple task. There are substantial differences in the authorized bachelor's degrees offered by nearly 2,000 American institutions (Podolsky and Smith, 1977). Although there are differences in formal designations, most bachelor's degrees indicate the successful completion of four years of general education with some measure of specialization as signified by majors and minors. The program must be prescribed, supervised, and evaluated by a departmentally based faculty willing to certify the degree's credibility. In order for institutions to award "accredited" degrees, they must meet certain governmental and association (voluntary) standards for prescribing requirements for the baccalaureate.

There are several types of bachelor's degrees. The traditional degree, the Bachelor of Arts, is principally characterized by the liberal or general nature of the educational requirements. There are professional bachelor's degrees in fields such as education, social work, and engineering. There are professional bachelor's degrees specially designed to meet the entry requirements of professional schools of law, medicine, and dentistry among others. However, the hallmarks of practically all bachelor's degrees, whether they represent highly specialized professional education programs or the broadest-based liberal arts general education, are that they require four years of study or its equivalent (usually expressed as 124 semester credit hours) and that they are considered to be a prerequisite for any advanced study, whether academic or professional.

Bachelor's degrees are often associated with the entry requirements for many occupations. Teaching at the common schools level, for example, requires the completion of a baccalaureate degree with certain requirements in the field of teacher education. Entry to this profession is also controlled by public agencies, since teaching certificates, awarded by licensing agencies, not institutions of higher education, are required for teaching in most accredited common schools. There are many other fields of endeavor that require the bachelor's degree as the entry credential. In most cases, these fields specify the type of educational preparation required and thus influence the curriculum design and graduation requirements for a given degree.

Many professions require the completion of a licensure examination in order to assure competence before entering a given profession. The bachelor's degree is typically prerequisite to taking many professional licensure examinations.

## Master's Degrees

Master's degrees represent the further proliferation of the idea of a broad diversity of degree levels. In many cases the master's is merely a continuation of the curriculum prescribed for the baccalaureate only at a more specialized level. For many fields, the master's degree has become the required credential for entry-level positions, thus succeeding the bachelor's degree as the major prerequisite. The master's represents the completion of advanced study beyond the bachelor's of one or two academic years (30 to 60 semester hours). In most cases, master's degrees represent a higher scholarly level of achievement, although in some instances, persistence and further experiential education rather than scholarly rigor are required.

There are two generally accepted categories of master's degrees in American higher education (Spurr, 1970). There is the traditional Master of Arts or Master of Science, which signifies the completion of a program of liberal studies, and there are a multitude of professional and field-related master's degrees designated by such titles as Master of Science in Teaching, Master of Business Administration, Master of Music. As Spurr (1970) states, "While nomenclature for the master's degree presents similar problems to that for the baccalaureate, it is even more complex and chaotic" (p. 65). The accepted distinction between the usage of differing degree designations provided by the Council of Graduate Schools in the United States is that the Master of Arts or the Master of Science without a specific field designation is to be used for "scholarly and teaching-oriented" programs (Spurr, 1970), while the professionally oriented degrees should carry some designation identifying the specific profession or field associated with the degree (e.g., Master of Gerontology).

## Intermediate Graduate Degrees

The intermediate level degree, such as the Specialist in Education, is a truly American phenomenon. This degree level, considered to fall somewhere between the master's and the traditional academic doctorate, is an attempt on the part of higher educators to provide a credential representing post-master's study without the sometimes perceived superfluousness of doctoral research (however, some would suggest that the intermediate degree is most appropriately viewed as a consolation prize awarded to those who cannot complete the doctorate rather than as a viable degree option). Spurr (1970) describes the intermediate degree as equivalent to the first phase of the doctorate marked by the completion of required course work and comprehensive examination but lacking the required research project. The "A.B.D." (all-but-dissertation) stage of the doctorate has gradually been replaced by formal designations such as Master of Philosophy or Candidate in Philosophy. On occasion, the Doctor of Arts is viewed as an intermediate credential. There are other forms of intermediate credentials, not formally designated as degrees, which do signify the completion of a stage of educational achievement somewhere between the master's and the doctorate. These credentials are most often labeled Professional Diploma, Certificate for Advanced Study, or Professional Certificate (Spurr, 1970).

## Doctoral Degrees

The highest credential in American higher education is the doctorate. This degree level, more than any other, has been subjected to scrutiny and discussion regarding the most appropriate requirements and designations. While probably too simple a definition for some, there are essentially three types of doctorates available in this country at the present time: academic discipline or field-based Ph.D.; applied doctorates; and professional doctorates. The academic Ph.D. represents for many the highest level of academic achievement. This degree, founded in the tradition of European universities, represents the rigor of advanced study and the demonstration of proficiency in independent research. The Ph.D. is viewed as the ultimate requirement for admission to the professoriate in most colleges and universities. This degree is criticized by others as an award for exercising the extreme in microeducational practice and having limited usefulness in the "real world." The Ph.D. represents advanced academic work beyond the master's degree and is usually described as requiring 90 semester hours beyond the baccalaureate. Although there is no standard time limit placed on completing the Ph.D., Spurr (1970) suggests that an average of five years is needed beyond the bachelor's degree to achieve a doctorate.

Applied doctorates represent the attempt of educators to develop a viable alternative to the research rigor traditionally associated with the Ph.D. Applied doctorates are extensions of advanced study in many fields that offer applied Master's degrees. Fields such

as business administration (D.B.A.), public health (Dr.P.H.), education (Ed.D.), and social work (D.S.W.) have developed alternative
degrees to the Ph.D. for persons wishing to achieve an advanced
level of education without pursuing the research rigor and skills
necessary for accomplishing the Ph.D. Although some would suggest
that applied degrees have a lower status than the Ph.D., there is such
an uneven quality among institutional requirements for all doctorates that any attempt at comparison is impossible. The primary
differences between Ph.D. programs and those for applied doctorates is the reduction in emphasis on empirically derived independent
research experience and the elimination of the oft present foreign
language requirements.

The professional doctorates represented by practitioner degrees
in law, dentistry, veterinary medicine, and medicine are different in
many respects from the "academic" doctorates. These programs are
seldom concerned with the accumulation of credit hours but attempt
to develop a set of refined practitioner skills necessary in the specific
profession. In the case of medicine, three or four years is required
beyond the bachelor's degree, which is not always expected before
admission. An essential part of medically related doctorates (including the D.D.S.) is an extended experience in using laboratory and
classroom knowledge. Specialization beyond the "first professional"
degree level is, in most cases, a possibility for professional doctorate
holders. These specializations represent a focus on some more narrowly defined subdivision of the profession rather than on advanced
study of the discipline or field, as is the case with an M.S. or M.A.

## Credentials in Gerontology Education

Credentials in gerontology education, reflective of the total higher
education scene, display much confusion and disarray. There are all
types of certificates and degrees available for persons wishing to
complete a credentialed program of study in gerontology. These
credentials lack any consistency in quality or composition, much to
the chagrin of leaders in the gerontology education field. The authors, in compiling data regarding credentials in gerontology education for the 1976–77 academic year, found that there were nine
alternative credentials available in gerontology education (Bolton,
1978). These credentials included a wide range of diversity, with
many being degree (Bachelor's and Master's) oriented or focused on
the provision of traditionally designated majors and minors for these

degrees. Certificates of specialization and concentration also represented a credential form for gerontology education.

## Associate's Degree in Gerontology

The associate's degree in gerontology is a recent development of American community or junior colleges. Terminal associate's degrees in gerontology are most often related to established fields that require some post-secondary training, e.g., the allied health professions and, in a very few cases, social work technologies. Explanations of the various degrees available at this level are found in Porter (1978), Tift (1978), and Cowley and Porter (1978). Ridley (1975) found that in 31 community or junior colleges in California offering gerontology instruction, Nursing Home Administration, Food Handling, Nursing Assistants, and Recreation Aides were the most common. One example of a formalized associate's degree program comes from Wayne Community College, Goldsboro, North Carolina (Crowley and Porter, 1978). This two-year Associate of Applied Science degree provides for a concentration in human services technology with an emphasis in geriatrics. Nursing home administration is another field in which applied associate's degrees have become increasingly important, and several states now require this level of educational attainment prior to licensure in the nursing home industry.

There is only a scattering of gerontology programs for transfer-oriented students at the community or junior college level. One such program at Riverside City College (California) represents an attempt to combine the principles of terminal and transfer programs at the junior college level while maintaining a clear focus on a core concentration in gerontology. The Riverside program (Bolton, 1978) may be viewed as a mini-version of many four-year undergraduate programs. It is placed in a division of social sciences (divisions are often used in community or junior colleges rather than the traditional departments) and incorporates the general education requirements of the college as well as a core of gerontology courses. The credential is viewed as preparation for enrollment in a bachelor's degree program or as a free-standing credential for employment at the paraprofessional level.

As the associate's degree in gerontology gains recognition as the first step in a career ladder of gerontologic occupations, community and junior college interest is being stimulated, as is the demand for persons with some post-high school training in gerontology, especially in urban areas with high concentrations of elderly persons. At the present time, some persons completing an associate's degree with an emphasis in gerontology are having difficulty finding jobs that meet their expectations for salary and responsibility. Although employers seem anxious to hire paraprofessionals with gerontology background, they are often unwilling to pay salaries higher than those paid to personnel who have little or no educational preparation. Before undertaking a major gerontology education program at the community or junior college level, program planners should first assess the marketability of the terminal associate's degree in the college's immediate area.

## Bachelor's Degree in Gerontology

Bachelor's degrees with some form of emphasis in gerontology have been available for nearly ten years. Degrees at the baccalaureate level are usually variations of either the standard general education, the Bachelor of Arts, or the professional development degrees. The few liberal arts programs are offered primarily by four-year private colleges and have traditionally focused on general as opposed to specialized educational programming. These institutions award the Bachelor of Arts with a major concentration in gerontology and attempt to maintain a curriculum with a balanced overview of the field of aging. The professionally oriented programs, on the other hand, tend to carry a specialized emphasis on aging in conjunction with professional occupational fields. These programs and their associated degrees prepare baccalaureate students for jobs in the nursing home industry, social-work-related occupations, and work roles connected with the aging network (Area Agencies on Aging, State Commissions on Aging, etc.).

The bachelor's degree has become popular in recent years because it provides institutional legitimacy. Awarding a degree is a significant measure of successful institutionalization of a program, indicating an enhanced ability to compete with traditional departments for resources. While many program directors have seriously questioned the advisability of degree programs in gerontology, the necessity for institutional security has prompted establishment of departments in order to lay claim to institutional resources.

The question of intended student outcomes for bachelor's degree programs is in continual dispute in gerontology education. The value and meaning of a bachelor's degree is not clearly defined and the nature of the employment market for such credentials is still unclear. For many gerontology educators there is a concern that the depth of subject matter in gerontology is insufficient to structure a complete degree program composed of the 30 to 45 semester hours. This concern is, as discussed previously, often given secondary status when the question of institutional survival and popular notions of emerging professions is considered.

## Master's Degree in Gerontology

Gerontology master's degrees have been available for more than ten years from such well-established programs as the University of South Florida and North Texas State University. This degree holds the greatest potential for continued development and expansion of any of the current credentials and is almost universally viewed as a professional education credential for such areas as long-term-care administration, social work, public administration, counseling and guidance, and recreation leadership. In most instances the master's requires an additional 30 to 40 semester hours of work beyond the baccalaureate. Some critics would suggest that there is currently insufficient knowledge in the area to warrant a full-fledged degree. This concern, however, has been muted by the popularity of the emerging degree programs and by the searching of program planners for degrees to compensate for the decline of enrollment in traditional liberal arts programs.

The market for professional master's degrees in gerontology is still hazy. One of the perennial questions raised by federal agencies about gerontology education has been the availability of employment for graduates of distinct gerontology degree programs. This concern has direct implications for current and future levels of funding; if graduates do not find relevant positions, soft funding for degree programs may diminish significantly. Again, institutionalization through the creation of gerontology departments seems to be the conditioned response to assure continued funding. The advent of clearly specified occupational roles for "gerontologists" and the resulting requirement of a specific degree in gerontology for these positions seem remote at the present time. Gerontology educators appear more content to wring their hands than to compile data describing occupational roles and concomitant preparation requirements. Nevertheless, the master's degree, for the most part established by highly reputable institutions, is becoming a standard credential in gerontology education. This is a precedent worth ongoing attention.

## Doctoral Degree in Gerontology

There are no true doctoral programs in gerontology available at this time. While some aspiring educators argue that they offer a doctorate in which gerontology is related to an existing field, the fact remains that these programs are not gerontology degrees. For many observers, the major question related to the doctoral degree remains unresolved: Does gerontology sufficiently approximate a discipline to allow doctoral level study? The strict application of guidelines in the definition of disciplinary status—e.g., a well-documented research methodology, a complete taxonomy of knowledge, a basis for empirically derived theory—suggests that gerontology is not and probably cannot be promoted as a discipline worthy of awarding the research-based Ph.D. At best, the precedent established by the several programs now awarding applied master's degrees may be applied to the applied doctorate. It may become appropriate to consider planning for applied doctorates sometime in the foreseeable future, but given the current economic state of higher education, it would seem inadvisable and downright fiscally irresponsible to proliferate applied doctorates in gerontology during the next few years.

There are three useful categories of doctorates in America, two of which appear to have some relevance for gerontology. In addition, several alternatives to the strictly defined doctorate in gerontology warrant careful consideration. There has been some discussion of the development of a multidisciplinary doctorate that would combine the disciplinary strength of established fields with gerontology. This format is already available in a few highly reputable programs across the country. The credentials do not represent true doctorates in gerontology but do indicate a formidable amalgamation of pertinent associated fields with gerontology.

## Alternative Credentials in Gerontology

A number of credentialing systems currently employed in gerontology education offer program developers some powerful alternatives to traditional degrees. These credentials do not represent complete degree programs but rather indicate an abbreviated curriculum that culminates in a certificate of specialization or concentration, a minor, or a cognate in gerontology.

Certificate programs in gerontology represent the oldest form of credential available for the field. Certificates are most often professional-education oriented and require field placements, internships, or practica in conjunction with upwards of 15 semester hours of course work. Certificate programs are available at all levels of higher education from the community or junior college to doctoral and postdoctoral programs in aging. The hallmark of this credential, whether designated as a specialization or a concentration (for these are typically synonymous terms), is that the amount of credit instruction appears to offer reasonable breadth and depth of subject matter on aging. There has been a wide variety of courses developed in gerontology (one recent survey generated some 25 typewritten pages of different course titles); however, there is a great deal of overlap in course titles and content. This overlap reveals a lack of content depth, which is the primary reason most gerontology educators give for preferring the certificate or similar credential to degree programs.

Minors and cognates are alternatives to degrees which are very similar in content and credit requirements to certificate programs. The difference among these three designations is the form the credential takes when awarded. Minors and cognates are usually noted on a student's transcript, with little other formal recognition given. The certificate, on the other hand, is generally presented as a formal "diploma," signifying the completion of a course of study. Differences are often evident in the way minors or cognates are administered and the manner in which certificate programs are carried out. The typical certificate is awarded by an identifiable gerontology education unit where admissions, program requirements, and evaluation measures are under the close supervision of the gerontology education faculty. In the case of minors or cognates, the faculty advisor in the major field may prescribe the program.

## Credentials, Structures, and Outcomes

Extensive interrelationships exist among the various aspects of gerontology education, for example, between credentials and the organizational structures developed. Moreover, the desired outcomes have a great effect on the structure of a given educational program; the choice of a degree rather than a certificate means that some outcome expectations are more appropriate than others. There is little empirical or substantiated evidence to indicate which combination of these variables constitutes the most defensible gerontology education program.

The alternatives to degrees (credentials, minors, and cognates) require limited institutionalization and a less prominent educational outcome: Minors and cognates can be offered by a small number of faculty serving primary fields and disciplines in addition to gerontology. Departmental subunits are all that is necessary for sustaining an ongoing certificate, concentration, specialization, minor, or cognate program; thus the cost, commitment, and developmental steps are held to a minimum. On the other hand, there are few data to indicate that this informal approach to gerontology education provides sufficient depth or credibility to give the graduate any advantage in the job market.

The intended outcomes for baccalaureate, master's, or doctoral degree programs in gerontology are generally lacking in specificity. While many degree programs recruit large numbers of students, evidence of successful student employment or long-term occupational progress of persons holding these degrees is only beginning to accumulate. The department/degree organization represents an attempt to institutionalize gerontology within higher education. The question of institutional security as the basis for choices regarding credentials, outcomes, and structures is quite inappropriate; disciplines are not created in response to a need for stable curricula and faculty positions. It is imperative that a solid case be made for credentials, structures, and outcomes based on empirical knowledge, educational needs, and applicability outside the educational institution. At the present time, this case has not been made clearly and logically enough to be persuasive to most gerontology educators.

Any assessment or discussion of gerontology education ultimately focuses on the one primary issue: whether the outcomes, goals, structures, and educational philosophy are most appropriately and effectively certified through a formal, distinct credential (degree) or through a less formal, alternative credential (minor, certificate). There is little evidence upon which to base a decision. More often than not, any discussion becomes a reflection of philosophical and emotional positions rather than a data-based examination of alternatives.

Inference from current practice suggests that a liberal arts program in gerontology warrants the awarding of the baccalaureate degree. There is great breadth to the field and a general understanding of aging within this culture and others can be gained through examination of the various processes and results of aging. This liberal education credential would signify a general familiarity with the area but would not necessarily prepare the graduate for any particular occupational role. There are well-developed curricula for master's degrees in applied gerontology in several highly reputable institutions. These programs are professionally oriented and prepare the students for social service or housing administration. Graduates have found employment in appropriate areas; however, continued expansion or proliferation of degree programs at the master's level may lead to oversupply of the market unless changes occur in job descriptions and educational requirements. Doctoral degrees are likely to begin appearing soon as the inevitable journey to the heights of academe is completed. Programs stressing scientific gerontology at the Ph.D. level are likely to depend upon one or more of the existing disciplines for depth of concepts and empirical data. Nonetheless, separate doctoral programs are now being discussed informally by many program builders, and it appears that the first of them will be initiated in the near future.

## References

Bolton, C. R. *Gerontology Education in the United States.* Omaha, Neb.: University of Nebraska at Omaha, 1978.

Cowley, D., and B. Porter. Design and Implementation of an Associate Degree Geriatrics Curriculum. Paper presented for Annual Meeting of the Association for Gerontology in Higher Education. Dallas, Tex., April 1978.

Podolsky, A., and C. R. Smith. *Education Directory: Colleges and Universities.* Washington, D.C.: U.S. Government Printing Office, 1977.

Porter, B. *Associate of Applied Science Degree in Geriatrics Technology.* Goldsboro, N.C.: Wayne Community College, 1978.

Ridley, J. H. *California Higher Education Study for the Aging: Community College Report.* Riverside City College, Riverside, Calif., 1975 (mimeo).

Rudolph, F. *The American College and University.* New York: Random House, 1962.

Spurr, S. H. *Academic Degree Structures: Innovative Approaches.* New York: McGraw-Hill, 1970.

Stewart, C. The Place of Higher Education in a Changing Society. In Sanford, N. (ed.). *The American College.* New York: John Wiley and Sons, 1967, pp. 894–939.

Tift, J. C. Considerations in Planning and Developing Certificate and Associate Degree Programs in Aging in Two Year Colleges. Paper presented for Annual Meeting of the Association for Gerontology in Higher Education. Dallas, Tex., April 1978.

# 8

# Curriculum in Gerontology Education

Curriculum for gerontology in higher education presents a fundamental problem for those considering the development of a program of study in the field of aging. From the foundation established for curricula by the liberal arts in Colonial American colleges to present-day career training programs focused exclusively on professional education, a broad spectrum of expectations have been fostered in an attempt to devise the "comprehensive" course of study. For many, curriculum development in higher education revolves around planning and conducting courses and programs of study that provide students with a coherent body of knowledge and skills. For others, curriculum centers on the organization of theoretical knowledge into the framework of the historically defined disciplines and professional fields. Thus, the evolution and refinement of curriculum may be perceived in distinctly different ways.

Nor should one assume that any curriculum is final or static. We can witness a contemporary movement to return to a highly structured "whole man" education and away from the occupational/vocational emphasis that has dominated recent times. It should be clear that curriculum does not remain in a steady state for long, but that continual evolution reflects the dynamism of American higher education. This continual ebb and flow of curricular theory presents problems for the program planner in gerontology, who must search for the appropriate balance between the practical and the expectation that what is learned must endure.

## Gerontology Curriculum Development

Gerontology education has been a subject for study in higher education for several years. During this period little consensus has developed regarding the most appropriate credentialing and curriculum structures for the varying needs of the field. Johnson (1967) has suggested two divergent purposes of curriculum: (1) to prepare persons to perform practical and prescribed duties for the clientele in the field they serve, and (2) to define a field of investigation that will further the boundaries of human understanding in order to facilitate the "greater good" of mankind. These divergent curricular views are most readily identified as a professional orientation and a liberal/ scientific orientation.

Johnson suggested that the distinction is between the concepts of "training" and "education." According to his definitions, the training curriculum is based upon practical considerations, acquiring information, skills, and attitudes for the performance of specified tasks in predictable situations. A curriculum for educational purposes, on the other hand, includes systematic learning experiences based upon the existing disciplines, which provide the general understanding necessary for association and interpretation of experience in unspecified, unpredictable situations. Thus, a distinction is made between two conflicting orientations of curriculum in the modern college and university—a distinction at the heart of the disagreement over gerontology curriculum.

Given this basic disagreement on the purposes of curriculum, the remainder of this chapter will examine three curricular patterns that dominate the field of gerontology education: (1) a liberal/general education orientation; (2) a professional school approach; and (3) a scientific or disciplinary-based emphasis. This chapter will not prescribe the courses to be included in a given program or the organizational structure to be developed. These programmatic aspects of gerontology education will be treated in detail in Chapters 10 and 11.

### Liberal/General Education Curricula in Gerontology

This model for curriculum development in gerontology education has as its intended outcome the provision of general liberal education experiences for the undergraduate and graduate student. Its primary purpose is to allow the student to develop a broad-based understanding of the sociological, psychological, and physiological processes of aging. The program of study would characteristically include modest concern for the mastery of content but would focus primarily on the students' personal development at the chosen level of higher education. There would be limited curriculum emphasis on the integration and sequencing of learning experiences; courses composing a given student's program would be based upon that individual's interests and educational needs. The program would likely be flexible and adaptable to the individual, rather than prescribed and authoritarian in nature. The liberalizing qualities of the content would take precedence over the vocational utility of the subjects, and the principal concern would be for breadth of understanding and knowledge of several aspects of gerontology content. The philosophical orientation in this type of curricular model would be relativistic and would allow students to seek courses consistent with their overall program of study.

An undergraduate curriculum based on this model would include course content in a variety of gerontological areas. These might include topics in the biological processes that cause aging; the physical changes typical at different life stages; the effects of reduced acuity in the perceptual abilities of the older person; intellectual changes such as motivation, rigidity, and learning over the life span; personality development; social and personal losses; social role adjustments; measures of life quality; cross-cultural variations in the aging processes; contemporary values affecting the old; historical roles of the aged; community organizations to meet the needs of older people; government programs for the aged; and personal interactions with individuals who are old. This curriculum would not emphasize the practical outcomes or employment opportunities in gerontology but would reflect the ideals, values, knowledge, understanding, and attitudes associated with the academic study of gerontology.

This type of gerontology program includes the content of most departments in the institution. Thus, courses are likely to be scattered through the whole college or university. The breadth and complexity of the content indicates that not all of these areas can be covered through the creation of new courses. Many will necessarily be initiated as units within existing courses and will be expanded or emphasized as student and institutional interest in the area develops. The underlying orientation to the content of aging is to incorporate that stage of life and its conditions into the existing framework of the liberal curriculum in such a way that age becomes another of the many facets of man studied in whatever subject is under consideration, without age per se being the principal focus.

This model of gerontology curriculum would most likely be employed in an undergraduate, baccalaureate program in which the entire course of study was focused on "whole person" development for general/liberal education reasons. Students attending liberal arts colleges that stress general/liberal education ideals would find this model most applicable. Community or junior colleges emphasizing transfer programs in the arts and sciences could employ this model, as could graduate level programs providing an academic cognate. Colleges and universities wishing to establish an academic support area in gerontology, but not wishing to put into place a full curriculum, would be best advised to consider the potential of adopting a liberal education model in building their institution's capability in gerontology. This approach, which focuses on the development of aging-related expertise by existing faculty specialists, offers a developmental process without exorbitant staff costs and the creation of several new listings in the college catalogue.

Students and faculty wishing to enter a program of studies offering a tangible career outcome or interested in either paraprofessional training or specialized graduate study would not consider this model applicable. It focuses on "making a life" rather than "making a living" and should be viewed in the career development sense only when combined with professional or scientific study in established practical fields or disciplines. This model is most useful in the institutional setting where a small offering of gerontology is most appropriate to the mission of the institution and the economics of curriculum expansion. The primary outcome for learners is understanding oneself and others rather than the practical application of what has been learned.

### Professional Education Curricula in Gerontology

There is little consistency among professional education programs between procedures (methodology) and purposes (philosophy) of education. These inconsistencies make it difficult to specify universally accepted characteristics of professional education generally or of gerontology education specifically. Therefore, the model presented for professional gerontology education program development will represent the writers' impressions of the "average" professional education approach to gerontology education. This average suggests a curricular balance among personal development, mastery of content, knowledge of the profession, and scholarly achievement and objectivity.

Professional education in practically all fields presents an overriding concern for problems, policies, and action as opposed to the abstractions, ideas, and theories of disciplinary-based curricula. The problem-centered professional education can be varied to allow alternative emphases, such as the preparation of policy experts concerned with national, regional, and local aging policy or caseworkers and counselors devoted to the problems of the individual elderly. But whatever specialized problems or focus a professional education curriculum in gerontology adopts, the emphasis is on career education as opposed to the general education approach just discussed. This career/vocational education emphasis does not suggest that professional education curricula lack rigor or scientific content. While there is an unspoken criticism of career education by some academic elitists, this criticism is most often unwarranted. Certainly some community or junior college curricula designed for the preparation of paraprofessionals have a strong "training" orientation rather than an "education" emphasis; the majority of two-year, four-year, and graduate professional curricula, however, represent sufficiently rigorous and theoretical study to provide the student with a solid education.

This content is likely to include background gerontology knowledge and skills that can be used in meeting the needs of the older person and understanding the service delivery system as it currently functions. Gerontology knowledge would probably include an overview of physical, psychological, and social aspects. In a sense, this portion of the curriculum would have great similarity to the liberal/general gerontology curriculum described earlier. It would, however, be much less broad and probably less deep as well. There would be a major emphasis on the development of conceptual understanding and skill development, with stress on the comprehension of several systems of human service, the awareness of one's own biases and fears, the development of techniques for working in an applied setting, the understanding of the planning and evaluation process, and the ability to choose and use several methodological approaches to working with clients and organizations. The professional curriculum would stress understanding the political and power environment in which practice and services are conducted, including the political process, the legislative effect on programs, the importance of funding, current community programs, needs of the community and specific populations, the role of professional associations, and means of determining the most effective approach to a given situation.

The professional education curriculum model for gerontology is appropriate at several levels of higher education, although it will result in different outcomes at different levels. For the community or junior college, the professional and paraprofessional outcomes reflect training for particular occupational roles, or, occasionally, for transfer to advanced educational programs, and thus stress specific curricular content and experiences. At the baccalaureate level the professional program of studies provides a broader-based general education sequence as well as the increased depth necessary for professional competence in performing occupational roles. At the postbaccalaureate level, professional education curricula show a greater emphasis on the skill aspects and a reduction in the general education components. Although some of the more established programs at this level have concentrated on the development of skills in a specific specialty area (e.g., North Texas State focuses on housing administration and planning), others have developed a more generic professional degree program not related to one specific set of vocational roles. These programs, offering applied degrees that purport to train "gerontologists," reflect a recent trend in training that gives credence to the idea that a specific role for a "gerontologist" is being established.

A number of professional roles appear to be developing, including employment in homes for the aging, state offices on aging, area agencies on aging, multipurpose senior centers, health and welfare agencies, and nursing homes. Much work is still to be done, however, on the classification, definition, and legitimization of these roles before a clear job market for master's degree graduates can be assured.

The growing awareness of the occupational opportunities for persons employed in aging-related agencies and institutions may, given the appropriate resource allocations, lead to professional roles for a variety of specialized gerontologists. This professional orientation to gerontology education allows the program developer to respond to regional or local employment needs, an essential element, according to Harris and Grede (1977), in the development of career education curricula. This model, then, is most appropriate for institutions with a commitment and available resources for establishing a curriculum in professional gerontology education which will provide sufficient didactic and field experience for the educational development of its students.

## Scientific Gerontology Education Curricula

The curriculum for a program of studies in scientific gerontology provides a third model of instructional orientation. Scientific or disciplinary gerontology is based upon the premise that knowledge has intrinsic value and its verification and expansion are a major purpose of higher education. This is manifested through an emphasis on methodology, hierarchy of knowledge, and a data base of verified, empirical findings. The student is socialized into a lifetime role of seeking the truth through a precise process of arriving at knowledge. This knowledge is expected to lead to the betterment of society and an improved quality of life for the individual. The emphasis is not on the identification and solution of social problems per se but on the development of knowledge which may incidentally be of use in addressing these problems. The instruction emphasizes depth in carefully prescribed areas in which the student and faculty member become experts in a restricted aspect of the world of knowledge and endeavor to expand this knowledge in the most appropriate directions.

Scientific gerontology curricula are likely to include two major components: (1) knowledge of the concepts and data currently verified and (2) skills in the use of methods and techniques to expand the knowledge in a defined area. The knowledge background would place an emphasis on the data that have been generated through empirical research and that impinge upon a narrow range of concerns. While this would include some of the same content as liberal/general gerontology, the purpose would be to gain a firm grasp of all of the research in a limited area. For instance, students interested in adjustment of persons in the later years would study the various factors that have been shown to affect adjustment: the importance of health, family, finances, roles, friends, and location; the part that self-concept and self-esteem play; the affect of the local subculture or ethnic group; the available support systems; the lifetime patterns of the individuals; and the historical experiences that distinguish this cohort.

In addition, the student seeking a scientific gerontology education would be expected to have skill in the use of research methods and instruments needed to expand the current state of knowledge. This would involve careful critique of other research, ability to use several data collection methods, knowledge of the strengths and weaknesses of the various instruments, familiarity with statistical techniques, ability to use computer facilities, skill in reporting the findings, and ability to acquire the extramural funding necessary for research undertakings.

Thus, scientific gerontology instruction would differ from professional instruction in its purpose, its depth, its breadth, and its outcomes. It would more likely be concentrated at the doctoral level and would typically lead to the production of researchers seeking the truth. It is distinct from liberal/general gerontology in that its depth is greater, its scope is narrower, and its outcomes are more empirically oriented. It is an attempt to provide the greatest depth and specificity possible; this is achieved only at the doctoral level.

## Conclusions

It has been suggested that curriculum theory for higher education is at best somewhat weak, and therefore the analysis and prescription of curriculum for gerontology education is difficult. The three models, liberal/general education, professional education, and scientific/disciplinary education, represent the majority of programmatic efforts presently being conducted across the country. These models reflect the intended student outcomes from participation in a given instructional program. The liberal/general curriculum model provides the knowledge necessary for a greater understanding of the basic aspects of aging as a stage of human development and in relation to other fields of general education such as psychology, sociology, and biology. The professional school model is career-education oriented with the focus being placed on problem solving and intervention practices. The scientific model provides depth of knowledge and skill in the generation of new knowledge; it is generally linked to doctoral education and is considered best placed when it is an adjunct to traditional disciplinary study.

## References

Harris, N.C., and J.F. Grede, *Career Education in Colleges*. San Francisco: Jossey-Bass, 1977.
Johnson, M. Definitions and Models in Curriculum Theory. *Educational Theory*, 1967, *17*, 127–140.

# 9

# Faculty Development In Gerontology Education

The term *faculty development* suggests that there are a series of processes available to faculty interested in acquiring competencies in the field of gerontology or in redirecting existing expertise for use in gerontology instruction. Since few current faculty members have had the opportunity to engage in any formal gerontology study, alternative approaches are needed to orient faculty and familiarize them with the content of this new field. Likewise, doctoral instruction designed to prepare college teachers must be modified to familiarize new faculty with the data and methods of gerontology.

Historically, college and university teaching faculty have been expected to hold an earned doctorate in an established discipline or professional field. To this requirement the additional expectation of significant, published research has been added in recent years. Although the primary function of most college faculty may be teaching, excellence in research has become the standard by which promotion and tenure decisions are made. The policies of "publish or perish" and "up or out" are no longer the exception but rather the rule.

There are three major factors that have directly influenced the current state of faculty development and preparation in American higher education. The first is a growing trend toward workshops and conferences designed to improve instruction. Mayhew (1977) suggests that faculty development directed toward the improvement of instruction started in the early 1970s, when instructional competence began to be measured by annual evaluations. Astin and associates (1974) suggest that the general decline in mobility of the professoriate and the increasing tenure density in many institutions or particular departments has the potential for encouraging faculty stagnation, especially in the area of instruction. The decline of faculty "nomadism" (Ashby, 1971) and the concomitant possibility of diminished motivation prompted college and university officials to become more discerning in awarding tenure and allowing teaching to remain an ancillary priority. The situation is not easily remedied, however, since most faculty realize that good teaching does not result in salary increases. As Richman and Farmer (1974) point out, "Teaching comes out badly in a typical professor's maximization criteria. Teaching minimizes, rather than maximizes, a professor's income" (p. 260).

A second factor effecting faculty development is closely related to the first—the anticipation of a steady state for higher education over the next 20 years, a state which is likely to be characterized by an aging faculty (Mayhew, 1977). The implications of an aging, stable, tenured faculty are tremendous. The traditional movement of faculty into and out of the main streams and branches of their professions and disciplines will decline as they become "set-in" at selected institutions. Tenured faculty will expect to teach those content areas in which they have interest and expertise. Those areas, however, may not be at all consistent with student demand. If there are no students to teach, what is the faculty member to do? Obviously, one remedy will be to develop some organized professional self-renewal so that faculty can "retool" in order to adjust their teaching specialties to the new, interdisciplinary fields that are forming.

A third factor in faculty development will be reduced demand for new faculty members over the next decade. Ashby (1971) suggests that at least two current faculty must retire or leave the institution in order for one new person to be hired. This low replacement ratio will have a marked effect on the availability of new positions and will likely mean that a greater number of faculty members will become localized in one institution. As loyalty to the local institution replaces loyalty to the discipline or profession, graduate enrollment may be expected to decline. This will occur as increasingly large numbers of faculty are retrained for internal positions; those who currently hold positions will not use the acquisition of an advanced degree to move to another institution. Rather, the retraining process of obtaining a few courses or workshops in the new area will replace enrollment in doctoral programs. This will result in reduced graduate program enrollments, which may produce dramatic effects on some universities.

Retraining of faculty, then, may become a major gerontology instructional undertaking, although some predoctoral instruction will continue. A number of specialized programs currently available at colleges and universities are designed to provide intensive and highly focused educational experiences for the professor wishing to reorient his/her disciplinary training and research emphasis toward the processes of aging. General education is available for faculty who wish to gain an overview of the field in order to include some gerontological content in their regular course offerings. Special seminars are offered for those who wish to move into gerontology programs, and opportunities are developing for predoctoral students to acquire an academic specialty related to gerontology, which may serve as the preparation for a future faculty role in a department or school. These alternative routes to faculty status in gerontology indicate the variance possible for "new" faculty members; how one becomes qualified as a scholar and teacher in the field of gerontology will depend on the intended role as well as the developmental route.

In gerontology, as in many other areas, the modal pattern for faculty development in the future will be through redirection of existing competence. This pattern will be especially prevalent in four-year colleges experiencing a shift in programmatic emphasis and in established universities attempting to adapt to new initiatives. Gerontology faculty are likely to be chosen from the proven scholars of other departments rather than being recruited from the crop of new doctorates seeking an entry position in higher education.

The various levels of higher education institutions must also be given consideration in any discussion of faculty development. These institutions require different types and amounts of faculty expertise and orientation. The instructor in the community or junior college would typically be less concerned about conducting and reporting highly specialized research than he would be with developing significant expertise in a practical field of endeavor and achieving effectiveness as a teacher. The professor in a liberal arts or four-year college would have a fairly specialized substantive educational background while not necessarily being expected to have a significant publication or research record. Teaching is paramount in a four-year or liberal arts college, while practical experience in a given field may or may not hold the utilitarian value given it in the community or junior college. The university professor engaged in training graduate students is expected to have a significant publications record to support his ability to conduct and report research; infrequently will he be required to have special competence as a classroom teacher.

The varying requirements for faculty at these several levels of higher education suggest that all faculty cannot be prepared in the same manner. To fill the specialized roles and missions of diverse institutions of American higher education, they will need differing skills, knowledge, and experience. Therefore, the next section will discuss alternative models for gerontology faculty development at four institutional levels: community or junior college, baccalaureate, master's, and doctoral.

## Gerontology Education Faculty Development

Within the four levels of higher education requiring different skills, there are curricular orientations that demand alternative modes of preparation. The following faculty orientations within levels will be described:

> Transfer-general education: community or junior college
> Terminal-career education: community or junior college
> Liberal-academic education: baccalaureate granting college
> Professional education: baccalaureate granting college
> Scientific-research education: master's granting college or university
> Professional education: master's granting college or university
> Scientific-research education: doctorate granting university

### Transfer-general Education:
### Community or Junior College

A general education program in a community or junior college is designed for transfer to baccalaureate degree granting colleges and universities and represents an academic orientation while maintaining a balanced focus on the purposes and intended learning outcomes associated with the institution. This focus is reflected in a gerontology curriculum designed to provide the learner with a broad-based understanding of the basic principles of adult development in the later years.

Faculty in this type of program would require, at the minimum, a master's degree in a traditional discipline or related field and substantive training in gerontology, or, of course, a master's degree from one of the newly organized programs in applied gerontology. Preparation for teaching in this setting requires a liberal educational philosophy with the whole-man outlook. Specialized content expertise or highly refined research skills probably would not be emphasized. Teaching skills and an understanding of a variety of instructional methodologies as well as an ability to establish rapport with students from diverse social and educational backgrounds would be essential characteristics. The ability to work with community organizations is a typical requirement for prospective community or junior college faculty as is the interest in providing service to the community. While this orientation does not stress the career education, because of the type of institution, faculty should understand and value career-vocational outcomes.

## Terminal-career Education: Community or Junior College

The career education movement, discussed in Chapter 8, represents the new frontier for gerontology education in the community or junior college. Programs have only recently begun to emerge to prepare "gerontology technicians" for paraprofessional and junior professional roles in the field of aging. These programs (it is not possible to keep track of current numbers as new ones are beginning constantly) focus on providing diplomas, certificates, and sometimes associate's degrees for persons aspiring to work in the local community or regional area. These undertakings have a strong vocational philosophy and often include at least as much experiential training as classroom learning.

A person wishing to develop faculty skills for this type of pro- *not so* gram would not necessarily have attained more than an associate's degree but would have had substantial work experience in the field. This experience builds the basis for supervising experiential learning as well as representing the content taught in courses. Only limited substantive academic preparation in gerontology or the liberal arts fields is required for this type of position. In many ways preparation for career community or junior college gerontology instruction resembles preparation for the research professor teaching doctoral students: The substance of the faculty member's academic career is merely a basis for the development of applied skills in performing the work at hand. For both, there is little emphasis placed on teaching competence or training, although for the community or junior college teacher such competence would carry significantly more weight; the greatest emphasis is placed on the person's "track record" in the application of his/her skill. A working knowledge of entry level positions within the aging network and the duties and competencies required for these positions would constitute a valuable portion of the aspiring faculty member's expertise. In order to develop coherent and comprehensive field experiences for students, the instructor would also need to be able to develop a strong liaison with local and regional agencies serving the elderly population.

### Liberal-academic Education:
### Baccalaureate Granting Colleges

Liberal gerontology education focuses on general educational experiences that provide students with a broad-based understanding of aging in relation to man's world. Faculty providing this type of instruction are typically committed to a value-oriented education rather than one that emphasizes specialized or applied experiences. They are likely to be content generalists having an educational background in the traditional disciplines or scholarly fields. They typically would not place a heavy emphasis on research or publication but would seek to integrate the great ideas of the past and apply them to contemporary issues and problems. Faculty for this type of program will hold a terminal degree in a disciplinary area and should be highly skilled at motivating and enlightening undergraduate students.

An appropriate means of attracting and training faculty for this type of program is to identify persons in departments experiencing enrollment declines and allow them to adapt their competencies to the field of gerontology. For those fortunate institutions having resources for leaves of absence, or for those institutions able to secure external funding for gerontology curriculum planning, there are numerous opportunities for faculty development. Many of the established gerontology education programs such as those at University of Michigan, University of Southern California, Syracuse, Pennsylvania State University, and North Texas State offer special summer workshops designed specifically for faculty development. These programs include one- and two-week sessions on general topics in gerontology as well as specific instruction in curriculum development and teaching resources. They are oriented to the part-time or casual learner rather than the full-time graduate student, thus providing busy faculty members a brief learning experience adapted to their summer schedule.

### Professional Education:
### Baccalaureate Granting Colleges

Professional gerontology education, by the nature of its curricular organization and intended mission, allows for several alternative faculty development approaches. For baccalaureate professional education programs, faculty preparation does not demand the extent of sophistication required of the graduate levels, although many of the characteristics of professionalism are similar. Gerontology education of this type concentrates on the skills and knowledge provided by higher education that will equip graduates for successful entry into a profession in the field of aging. The faculty in this type of program have several alternative preparatory routes. Some acquire substantial professional work experience and then complete an applied master's or doctorate in order to meet institutional requirements. Others obtain an applied or disciplinary master's degree and then work in professional service positions before accepting a teaching assignment. A third category may have limited experience in the professional setting, relying on intermittent consulting and a terminal degree from an established professional school for their practical orientation. The key to preparation for instructional roles of this type and level is a professional orientation reflected in substantial applied experience or substantive university training.

### Scientific-research Education: Master's Granting College or University

The primary function for faculty involved in scientific gerontology education is to teach fundamental principles and methodology for research. At the master's degree level, the orientation is very similar to that of transfer programs at the community or junior college level. The primary focus is on preparing students for more sophisticated learning experiences — in this case, doctoral programs. Although this outcome is primary, many graduates of master's degree programs do not pursue doctoral study; rather they seek teaching positions in four-year colleges or secure employment that requires narrowly defined study.

One common avenue for securing a faculty position in a scientific gerontology education program is the completion of a Ph. D. in an established discipline in addition to substantial content in aging. The dissertation would focus on the processes of aging within the bounds of the discipline. This approach allows the fortunate few so trained to pursue positions in major, research-oriented gerontology education programs. However, obtaining such a position often involves more luck and political savvy than true methodological or content expertise.

A second route to faculty status would involve transfer from an existing position in a related academic field, typically preceded by the completion of postdoctoral study in gerontology. Many major universities appear to prefer this staffing approach to hiring junior faculty to build a program. Through a postdoctoral program of a major university or a sabbatical year of research and intensive study in gerontology, an established researcher can acquire the content and methodological competence necessary for a faculty role in a scientific gerontology program.

### Professional Education:
### Master's Granting College or University

As with other levels, professional gerontology education at the master's level requires an emphasis on practical applied experience. Since this type of program is popular nationally, the need for faculty prepared in the practical aspects of service delivery continues to grow. Although many faculty members teaching graduate professional education have had substantial community work experience, this is not an absolute requirement for instructional positions. Many faculty with fundamental academic training in the traditional disciplines are needed in order to provide the theoretical bases for understanding human behavior and service delivery. Thus, there is a need for two kinds of faculty in professional graduate programs, the balance between these two types depending upon the general orientation of a given program.

Faculty with practical experience as their principal expertise will also be expected to have a solid academic foundation in order to provide the conceptual understandings for effective service delivery. A terminal degree is a requirement of most present-day graduate programs; therefore, faculty would need to have completed a doctorate in either an applied social science or a professional field and be able to teach in a conscientious and effective manner.

### Scientific-research Education:
### Doctorate Granting University

Once the highest level of academe is reached, the development of faculty for instructional roles offers few variations. The faculty in scientifically oriented doctoral programs must demonstrate a high level of scholarly productivity and a history of teaching and research success, and the professor in an applied doctoral program cannot expect to have a significantly different record of achievement. There may be instances where a truly outstanding public servant with a long history of successful executive experience will become a faculty member of a major doctoral degree granting program. However,

only in these rare cases is the terminal Ph. D. not a minimum requirement for gaining faculty appointment. The research scientist/profes-
sor is the hallmark of prestigious graduate institutions, and it matters
little whether students in this setting are pursuing an applied or a
scientific doctorate. In most cases the only difference between the
applied doctorate and the research-based doctorate is the requirement for research tools. The nature of the dissertation may vary,
although this difference has become blurred as the prestige of one
degree or the other waxes and wanes.

Faculty development in doctoral programs is a process of attaining a highly scientific terminal degree, climbing the ladder of academe through the succession of available ranks, and producing a
publications record of substantial size. These requirements are standard for the scientific-research oriented faculty member and differ
only in the possible substitution of outstanding consultative services
for the faculty in applied programs.

## Current Faculty in Gerontology Education

In a study conducted by Bolton et al. (1978) and described in greater
detail in Chapter 6, 402 universities, colleges, and community colleges were surveyed to ascertain, among other things, the characteristics of faculty involved in gerontology instruction. The data
collected in that survey support the contention that many faculty
paths to gerontology exist. The data provide some insight into the
characteristics of faculty in the major programs of this country in
1977.

Faculty members in gerontology education programs were
asked to designate their primary academic assignments. Approximately 16 percent indicated that they were located in a gerontology
unit, 13 percent in sociology, 11 percent in health professions, 10
percent in education, nearly 10 percent in psychology, and 7 percent
in social work. The remaining 32 percent were distributed among
other areas such as social science, human development, behavioral
science, public service technology, English, human services technology, biological science, and community service. Thus, gerontology
units had the largest number of faculty ($n = 64$), but the remaining
333 were widely distributed among 21 other departmental designations.

Most faculty members in gerontology have been involved in this
field for a relatively short period of time. The mean number of years

of gerontology teaching was 4.7 for the whole sample, with 20 percent having been involved one year or less, and 35 percent less than three years. The longest tenure was held by an individual who indicated that he had been involved in gerontology instruction for 29 years—clearly one of the founding fathers of the field. Similarly, most of the instructors devote a minority of their time to gerontology. The average faculty member taught less than one gerontology course per semester or term, and only 15 percent taught as many as three courses in gerontology per term. The faculty then are fairly recent recruits to the field and spend only a portion of their time in this area of instruction.

Nearly all of the faculty members responding to the survey held graduate degrees; approximately two-thirds had attained the doctorate and most of the remainder held the master's degree. Only 3 percent indicated a professional degree, such as in law or medicine. More than half of the faculty completed their highest degree since 1970, and 10 percent had completed it within the last 12 months. Thus, the faculty primarily represent the young and less-experienced portion of the professoriate. This conclusion is supported by an examination of the academic ranks they hold. Thirty-three percent of the respondents held the rank of assistant professor, 28 percent were associates, and 27 percent were full professors; nearly 12 percent held the title of instructor or lecturer. Fifty-seven percent were male and 43 percent were female.

The conclusion that current gerontology faculty are somewhat less mature than those of many traditional areas is also supported by the number of publications reported. Of the 192 faculty who claimed to have any publications at all, the mean for the field of gerontology was 7.9, while 9.8 were claimed in other academic areas. Although there is no way of assessing the quality of these articles or the journals in which they appeared, it can be speculated that faculty in gerontology are producing publications at only a modest level, especially when one considers that nearly half of the faculty claimed no publications whatsoever.

The picture of the current gerontology faculty member, then, is one of a fairly young person who has a degree in another disciplinary or professional area and who has moved into gerontology instruction in the past four or five years. Instruction is being supported by publications both in gerontology and in the disciplinary area, and teaching assignments remain divided between the two fields. Probably some self-education and participation in conferences and workshops has assisted the individual in preparing for the change in focus, but there are no specific data to support this assumption. In general, the picture emerges of a redirection of career as the opportunities in gerontology are presented to current faculty members.

## Administrator Development in Gerontology Education

An often overlooked role in the development of gerontology education is that of the program administrator. These positions are highly varied depending upon the nature and focus of a given institution's mission and intent for gerontology education. For the majority of programs, the position entails responsibilities comparable to that of a typical departmental chairperson. In others, the activities are broadened to include the facilitation of public service and the conduct of research. In these instances, program direction requires administrative skills and involvement well beyond those of the traditional department. No known programs are oriented primarily to the development of gerontology education administrators. While the possibility exists for aspiring administrators to pursue advanced work in higher education administration or in other related fields, the combination of substantive training in administration and gerontology is yet to be developed. The majority of current gerontology program directors have not had specific training in these areas, but this limitation does not appear to hinder their successful completion of that role.

Generally, department chairpersons in American colleges and universities hold the rank of professor in that discipline or field and have been promoted (some consider this a dubious honor) to chairperson because of their general competence, acceptability to the faculty, and willingness to supervise the operation of their department. This is also the case for gerontology education; however, extensive government and foundation funding support of gerontology education requires that most program administrators have a firm understanding of "grantsmanship" and federal funding procedures. In many emerging programs, the faculty member most interested in furthering the development of gerontology curricula becomes the administrator, thus assuming the position based upon interest rather than expertise or preparation.

A growing number of major centers and institutes of gerontology require more than a passing interest to administer. These positions (there are approximately nine such openings available at the time of this writing) require administrators with competencies in both substantive gerontology and administrative practice. This combination of skills is rare among most faculty. Probably the solution to the growing demand for skilled and knowledgeable administrators will be the development of in-service or sabbatical educational experiences by which gerontology education faculty can learn the unique qualities of their administration. This type of program, however, is not presently available.

There are a sufficient number of well-developed programs across the country that could supply administrative internships for faculty interested in career development of this type. For faculty in emerging programs, it might be best to avoid the largest centers such as University of Michigan, Duke, Syracuse, and University of Southern California, but rather to spend a few weeks to a semester in a well-developed, mid-sized program like Alabama, North Texas, University of South Florida, Nebraska, Utah, or Oregon. This exposure could prove to be very beneficial in developing a practical understanding of such programmatic aspects as grant support, curriculum development, community articulation, faculty development, library materials, student expectations, program organization, and administrative process. Although most administrators eventually master each of these areas, a great deal of time and effort might be saved through a planned internship experience.

## Gerontology Faculty Development in the Future: A Prospectus

It would appear that there is currently an adequate supply of faculty being trained in various aspects of gerontology to meet the demand. The advertisement of faculty positions is a relatively rare occurrence and administrative opportunities, although more widespread, are not great enough to cause a supply shortage. Qualified applicants are sometimes in short supply, but most positions do not go unfilled. Faculty are retrained or learn the requirements of these new positions on the job.

The greatest future demand for gerontology faculty is likely to be in the community or junior colleges and four-year, baccalaureate granting institutions. These potential positions arise from a growing interest in career training and general education in gerontology. As the smaller institutions become aware of the possibility of refocusing curricula and begin to seek trained "gerontologists" to develop new programs, the demand for faculty with substantive educational experience in gerontology will grow. One problem associated with this potential growth is the lack of qualified persons willing to work in the institutions most likely to need their services. The unique vocational mission of community or junior colleges and the teaching orientation of the small liberal arts colleges suggest that a new type of faculty member for gerontology will be in demand.

Future development of gerontology instruction in a growing number of colleges, community colleges, and universities is a very real possibility. Once adequate definitions for occupational roles in gerontology are accepted, and once a general pattern for instructional programs is established, the field could expand very rapidly. If this expansion does occur, the demand for additional gerontology faculty would likely grow substantially and the supply might well become inadequate. Although most current openings are for junior level positions, many seek faculty at the associate and full professor level. Recruitment of this type of faculty is difficult unless one is willing to accept a transfer from another disciplinary or professional area. There is now only a limited number of persons at these levels willing to move, making recruitment of senior faculty members to lead the programs very difficult.

Although speculative program development is generally discouraged in this time of "stable state" economics, the potential shortage of qualified faculty with special competencies demanded by community or junior colleges and baccalaureate granting institutions suggests the wisdom of planning for programs such as the multidisciplinary doctorate. In the long run, the demand for faculty in gerontology will never be as great as for other, larger fields, but it seems reasonable to expect most academic administrators to realize that aging/gerontology is an important part of any institution's curriculum, whether as a full program of study or as a few support courses for the established disciplines and professional programs, and to encourage its growth in the years ahead.

# References

Ashby, E. *Any Person, Any Study.* New York: McGraw-Hill, 1971.
Astin, A., and associates. *Faculty Development in a Time of Retrenchment.* New Rochelle, N.Y.: CHANGE Magazine Publications, 1974.

Bolton, Christopher R., Donna Z. Eden, Julia R. Holcomb, and Kathleen Ryan Sullivan. *Gerontology Education in the United States: A Research Report.* Omaha, Neb.: The Gerontology Program, University of Nebraska at Omaha, 1978.

Mayhew, L. B. *Legacy of The Seventies.* San Francisco: Jossey-Bass, 1977.

Richman, B. M., and R. N. Farmer. *Leadership, Goals, and Power in Higher Education.* San Francisco: Jossey-Bass, 1974.

# 10

# Development of Gerontology Education Programs

Educational programs in gerontology vary greatly in their purpose, breadth, organization, and intended educational outcomes. In order for faculty and administrators to develop a program of studies, it is necessary for them to define clearly a planning process that will assure that careful consideration is given to the numerous issues involved. Although many of these issues have been described in the preceding chapters, it is appropriate here to integrate them in order to provide an organized approach to program development. Thus, the individual program developer may use this chapter as a guide for the planning and implementation process.

The uniqueness of the local institution and the community it serves will greatly affect the planning of any educational program. The program developer will bring to the process a set of biases; the institution and academic unit will evidence certain programming priorities; constraints will be placed on the development of any new program; and the contemporary situation may suggest that more or less caution should be used in anticipating future resource allocations. These considerations will vary from one institution to another. We must assume in this chapter that we are dealing with a traditionally defined institution with a typical educational mission; the many variations cannot be taken into account here. Thus, the planning model presented is an idealized version of the development process. This idealization does not detract from the usefulness of the model but does suggest that it must be modified to include the primary local variables when applied to a specific institution.

Ten stages are included in the planning process presented here.

Although they are generally sequential, some of the stages overlap significantly. It is therefore necessary to consider the implications of some of the later stages before reaching a final decision on earlier ones. The stages are parts of the whole process in which each decision will affect all of the others. Since early decisions are likely to eliminate some options for later stages, a back-and-forth methodology is most appropriate in the actual process. In pursuing the planning process in this manner, the best programmatic emphasis is likely to evolve, with little conflict with the institutional mission.

## Stages of Planning Gerontology Education Programs

### Stage One: The Institutional Context

Any program of instruction must adhere to the general mission and goals of its sponsoring institution. Therefore, the first step of the planning process is to review the priorities, goals, programming limits, and emphases of the host institution. A small liberal arts college, for example, would likely emphasize general education at the undergraduate level; other types of instruction (e.g., vocational training) would be inappropriate. In a large public university, the mission may be very broad and allow the development of instruction at many levels, pursuing varying philosophies and operating through many organizational structures.

The review of the institutional context should include the identification of current and/or expected constraints that would interfere with the proposed program. For instance, the governing boards of several institutions have recently announced that they would approve no new degree programs. This obviously would eliminate one possibility for program development in gerontology. In other instances, statewide coordinating bodies have designated one institution as the principal offerer of gerontology education, so others are likely to experience difficulty in initiating programs in this area.

Another initial consideration in the assessment of the institutional context is the availability of resources for program operations. If the institution is experiencing financial difficulties, it is unlikely that money for gerontology could be made available internally. Some small, private colleges have attempted to save themselves from financial disaster by attracting more older students to campus, by remodeling dormitories for retirement housing, and by developing service programs for older people. The financial expectations for these programs are likely to place severe strains on the development of gerontology education since the generation of additional income for the institution is often a primary concern. Even when the situation is not critical, internal resources are likely to be needed to initiate a viable program, so the institution's financial situation is of great importance.

The institutional environment, then, sets the tone, defines the program planning parameters, and indicates the constraints within which the gerontology program must be planned, developed, and operated. It cannot be overemphasized that an understanding of institutional climate is crucial to the development of the program. Too many faculty and administrators have sought to replicate another institution's instructional program only to discover that its functions and mission were inappropriate for their context. Any program in a given field will vary from one institution to another, and the institutional uniqueness must be clearly understood before planning can be initiated.

## Stage Two: Current Gerontology Activity within the Institution

Most institutions of higher education already have some activities related to gerontology instruction. This activity may take the form of courses in gerontology, life-span development, medical ethics, service delivery systems, physiology, adult education, government processes and programs, health care, normal or abnormal psychology, family living, pensions and retirement benefits, employee retraining, or contemporary social problems. Other activities may include research in which faculty members are attempting to use age as one variable in a major study or where cross-generational samples are being employed. Similarly, services to the community may involve education of older people, field placements for students in community agencies, tuition reductions or waivers, gold card admissions to institutional programs and events, or a variety of other services or programs that are offered to older persons.

Existing activities may provide a base on which any additional program development can be built. By incorporating existing undertakings into the planned program, a smaller number of new courses will need to be developed, and faculty and student recruitment are facilitated. This consideration can save time, resources, committee work, and injured feelings. On the other hand, some current activities may have little relevance to the planned instructional program. For example, a developing doctoral concentration in gerontology may have little relation to existing undergraduate courses or community service programs. It is therefore important early in the planning process to learn not only what is already underway but its potential relationship to the planned program. Another obvious reason for an institutional inventory of current gerontology activity is the programmatic "turf" issue. If faculty or administrators are already involved in programs related to gerontology, they may hesitate to offer support to some other faculty member infringing on their territory.

Similarly, it is helpful to be aware of any current planning being contemplated or initiated which would relate to gerontology instruction. Although other efforts may not become reality for some time, if at all, it would be helpful to know, for instance, if a degree in human services was being planned in which gerontology might become a related concentration, or if an emphasis in long-term care was being proposed which might be incorporated into future planning.

Some institutions of higher education have assessed current programmatic activity in a questionable manner. They have identified several courses that include some gerontological content, simply listed these courses in one section of the college catalogue, and then asserted that they offer a gerontology curriculum. Although it is possible that some colleges and universities might have an existing series of courses needing only a coordinating mechanism, it is likely that curricular gaps will demand supplemental courses to form a comprehensive gerontology education program.

Regardless of the extent of the current gerontology education activity, much can be gained from a complete review of the situation. Potentially interfering structures, persons, or rules can be recognized; interested persons can be incorporated into future planning; available resources can be identified; and the current system can be better understood. Although we have emphasized an assessment of the programming of the host institution, the same case can be made for an inventory of local and regional programs and activities. If other colleges are already involved, if professional associations are active in continuing education, if nationally visible persons are local residents, it would be more than appropriate to know their current level of activity and to include both individuals and institutions in the planning process.

## Stage Three: Determination of Program Focus

There are numerous alternative approaches to curriculum development in gerontology education; some require much new effort, others very little. It is feasible for an educational institution simply to bring together existing courses in order to create a unified "program of instruction." It is also possible to modify a few existing courses in order to include additional gerontology content. Some gerontology education programs concentrate on the conduct of continuing education for practitioners through workshops or conferences. Others have developed limited formal course offerings but have created impressive field experience centers, which assist students in applying their classroom learning in community settings. An alternative to the modification of courses or the provision of field experiences in aging agencies and institutions is the development of an entirely new series of courses leading to the designation of a concentration, specialization, minor, major, or degree in gerontology.

The faculty and/or administrators responsible for planning a gerontology program may wish to consider any or all of these options as well as combinations of them. Because there are many alternatives, it is important that a decision on program emphasis be made as early as possible in the planning process. This initial focusing can eliminate least feasible choices, based upon institutional mission, resources, or preferences.

Although many programs incorporate several of the above alternatives, it is advisable to determine early in the planning process which are of primary importance and which are peripheral and to be developed only after the core program is well established. Too often, all of the options are exciting, and program planners fail to specify which are to be given lower priority. This typically results in a fragmented plan of questionable quality, with no identifiable programmatic strength.

In order to avoid this pitfall, several questions related to program design need to be addressed and at least tentatively answered. The first question is whether the course should be designed primarily for junior college, baccalaureate, master's, doctoral, or intermediate graduate level students. The answer to this question will depend upon the institution, the interest of the faculty and administrators involved, the desired outcomes, and the available resources. Many programs currently offer a single set of courses to undergraduate and graduate students simultaneously; this conserves resources but often leads to difficulties since graduate and undergraduate students have varied educational backgrounds, levels of academic expertise, and educational expectations.

A second question, that of program focus, would be addressed through the three dichotomies presented in Chapter 4. First, should the program of instruction emphasize content breadth or depth? The second dichotomy asks whether the program should be separate from other departments or academic units or whether it should function as an adjunct to an existing departmental entity. This answer will probably determine the type of organizational structure chosen as well as whether a free-standing degree or a concentration within an existing field is to be offered. The third dichotomy raises the question of educational outcomes, whether the program focus should be professional, disciplinary, or academic.

Chapter 11 will present three program models in which the differing outcomes are more completely described. At this point, it seems sufficient to suggest that these decisions, made early in the planning process, will be very helpful in focusing the instructional program, in determining which faculty members' contributions will be most relevant, in assessing the resources needed, and in eliminating many of the peripheral alternatives.

## Stage Four: Educational Program Outcomes

The determination of program emphasis is a major step in focusing the instructional program. However, greater specificity is needed to assure that the course content will result in the most desired student learning outcomes. These may be formulated in terms of student knowledge; practice or research skills; or attitudes, beliefs, and values the student should acquire. In order to assure program clarity, intended outcomes in each of these areas should be determined and specified.

One way to approach this process is to identify the goals or objectives of the instructional program. Although this is a common step, goal statements are often so general and lofty that they really do not eliminate many of the possible program impacts. What is needed is a method of reducing the scope of the goals envisioned and focusing more closely on a few selected outcomes. This focusing may be achieved by the identification of the desired characteristics of program graduates. For example, in a professionally oriented program, it might be possible to suggest that principal student learning outcomes should emphasize the delivery of social or health services to older people. Thus, the instruction would include the common problems facing contemporary older people, the organization of the community services for the aging, the techniques for planning and developing new services, and the methods of assessment and evaluation of services for the elderly. Identifying these or similar outcomes sets the direction for courses and field experiences.

In effect, this emphasis on intended outcomes would propose the type of students to be recruited and graduated. By emphasizing the focus of the program, it is possible to guide faculty in the development of curricula, in the establishment of field work experiences, in the setting of achievement standards, and in the placement of students upon their graduation.

## Stage Five: Course Development

Most gerontology program development will involve the creation of new courses or the modification of existing ones. This is often a tedious process involving large amounts of time dealing with department, college, and university committees which grant approval for new courses and revisions of the curriculum. However, it is of great importance that it be done well initially since changing the curriculum at a future point will consume additional resources and time.

If the appropriate decisions have been made in stage three, it will be clear whether the program will lead to a degree, a specialization, or a minor. This will determine the number of credit hours required for completion of the program, as well as whether the focus will be professional, academic, or disciplinary. The more specific decisions to be made in stage five include the number of new courses to be developed, the number and type of courses to be modified, the level of the courses, which courses will be required and which elective, objectives for each course, texts to be used, instructional methods to be employed, and the nature of the evaluation process.

In large part, the specific planning must be left in the hands of the individual faculty member teaching a given course. However, it generally proves valuable to provide each instructor with an understanding of the goals of the entire program in order to assure agreement of course emphasis and intended program outcomes. If left without this orientation, the faculty will often develop courses which may be completely defensible on individual merits but which will not conform to the intended focus and objectives of the program. For instance, a faculty member may decide to emphasize research methodology and findings for a course which had been anticipated to lead to professional practice outcomes. The result, although valuable, will be inappropriate to the intended objectives of the program.

Another consideration in the area of course development is student expectations. Since typical gerontology students are somewhat older than the mean and have some work experience or are currently employed, questions are often raised about credit for previous practical experiences. This experience may be assessed through the use of CLEP tests or may simply be legitimized by the award of some general education credit for work or life experience; the amount and type of credit needs to reflect institutional policies and program goals. Other questions arise in the scheduling of class sections. Employed students desire to take courses in the late afternoon or evening, but full-time students prefer morning or early afternoon classes. Not only does scheduling become a problem for older, experienced students, but some consideration of instructional methods for adult students may also be required. Older students often have a great deal of practical information to share, and a discussion or seminar format may prove superior to the more traditional lecture.

Off-campus courses also may provide an alternative approach. Many colleges and universities have found that personnel in area agencies on aging, state offices on aging, welfare departments, nursing homes, and other agencies and institutions working with the elderly may request that credit courses be offered in their place of work. This client group offers a substantial opportunity for increasing the impact of the gerontology instruction program, but it raises a number of problems in terms of admissions, scheduling, budgeting, staffing, library and other learning resources, and course content. The advantages, however, are generally agreed to outweigh the problems, and increasing numbers of programs of this type will be developed in the future. The decision to undertake modified program delivery is best made early in the program development process in order to facilitate cooperative planning, to assure a flexible course structure, and to anticipate the needs of a nontraditional student group.

## Stage Six: Field Experience and Practica

Gerontology instruction often includes planned exposure to older people in both the community and institutions or agencies that serve the elderly. This practical exposure is implemented through field experience, practica, field orientation, or other activities bearing a similar name which encourage students to leave the campus for direct exposure to the "real world." Professionally oriented instructional programs often require as much as a year of experience in an agency setting; liberal gerontology education would not emphasize field experience but would be likely to include visits to several agencies where students could gain an overview of the existing service programs.

There are many questions to be addressed in the planning of field instruction, the length and type of field placement being of primary concern. If the focus of the academic program is on preparing professional practitioners, the field work experience will be lengthy, providing experience in a single institutional or agency setting which is intended to socialize the student and offer an opportunity for role modeling. In a scientific gerontology program the practicum experience may not be undertaken in the field at all but rather in the laboratory operated by the educational institution. In this case the student would assist the senior faculty members in ongoing research projects relevant to the student's principal field of interest.

Another consideration in the development of field work is the student supervision that will be provided. Since a student is often placed in an institution or agency setting for a significant period of time, the quality of learning will be dependent upon the nature of the field organization and the type of student supervision provided. If the agency supervisor devotes adequate time and care to the practicum process, assuring that the student is well supervised, involved in an increasingly demanding series of experiences, and given the needed access to resources and personnel, the student will be able to grasp agency purposes quickly and assume a meaningful role in ongoing operations. Thus, the agency representative who supervises students in the field is the key to a successful field experience. Many agency personnel are unfamiliar with this role of field instructor, so care should be exercised in the selection and orientation of the field experience supervisor in order that the most beneficial results will accrue to both the participating student and the agency.

Other questions regarding practica relate to the integration of field work with classroom instruction. Since there is no automatic transfer of classroom knowledge to practice, many educational institutions offer a seminar concomitant with field work to allow students to compare experiences, receive guidance from faculty on difficult situations, broaden their understanding of the organization of services and programs of the community, and evaluate their progress as professionals. The practicum seminar is also an appropriate time to review the comprehensiveness of the community service system, to learn more about government funding and operation, and to hone interpersonal skills.

The field experience offers the possibility of combining the practical with the theoretical and adds a substantial instructional element to most gerontology education programs. Since gerontologists are often humanistically oriented, the practicum provides the opportunity for direct exposure to older persons, for modifying biases regarding the elderly, and for learning more about interpersonal relationships between the professional and the client. Planning for the field experience requires the identification of appropriate agencies, the determination of their requirements and limitations for student interns, the assessment of agency quality as a learning environment, and the development of agency commitment to participate in the educational process. This planning need not be difficult, since many practitioners attach some status to affiliation with university or college instructional programs, but arrangements should be initiated early in the planning process in order to obtain support and to give consideration to the concerns of the agency staff.

### Stage Seven: Development of Student Services

Decisions made on the type and structure of the gerontology instructional program will largely determine the extent of student services to be provided. A degree program will require many more student services than will a concentration or specialization program. However, in practically every case there will be the need for some staff time allocated for the provision of assistance in recruitment, admissions, academic advisement, and job placement. These services may be provided in a fairly informal and low-key manner, or they may require a great deal of a faculty member's time. Regardless, student services need to be carefully planned in order to assure their effective availability.

New instructional programs face the challenges of becoming known to their potential student constituency. Publicity, promotional materials, and contact with other faculty are required in order to assure that current and entering students know of the program's existence. Information may be directed toward students who are already attending the institution and who might be interested in enrolling in the new program or toward entering students who are still in the process of choosing their academic specialty. Analysis of current student bodies in many institutions has indicated that many registrants are already employed in community agencies and institutions oriented toward older people. These students have recognized a gap in their knowledge of gerontology and are attempting to remedy this through participation in formal education. Many program planners have utilized this awareness to recruit students from local service agencies and institutions.

Although currently employed students may be a readily available audience, program planners should not ignore the long-term potential of recruiting students from the current enrollees of the institution. Registrations may not come quickly from this group since additional time will be required to convey the meaning of gerontology and the value of instruction in the field of aging; however, continuing student enrollment is assured through the participation of full-time students. Program development that responds to the felt needs of current community services personnel may prove a transient solution to enrollments, but, too often, these persons are seeking answers to very specific and pressing questions that either can be answered quickly or are not addressed in normal course content. Once the practitioners' immediate concerns are met, it may be difficult for him/her to maintain interest in a conceptual or theoretical program.

The admissions process for nontraditional students (community practitioners) is often more complex than for traditional full-time students. Nontraditional students usually have been outside the college environment for several years, may have had spotty academic records, may be unfamiliar with the educational institution's bureaucratic procedures, and may wish to take only a course or two rather than enrolling in a regular degree program. In any case, they are likely to need help in the admissions and enrollment processes. Since their interest is on gerontology content rather than the entire educational program, they may be more resistant to institutional requirements and procedures and seek shortcuts to the standard admissions procedure. This results in a need for greater assistance from some member of the gerontology faculty or admissions office staff.

Academic advisement is an important function of any educational program. Since gerontology is often considered to be an adjunct to another degree program, it could be assumed that little academic advising would be necessary. This is not the case, however. The informal student information network often works poorly when students are not involved in a degree program. Students may know few other persons in their classes, so may require the formalized support and information that the advising process can provide.

Gerontology is a relatively new academic field; there is a limited amount of general information in most institutions about the expectations and results of such instruction. Consequently, faculty time needs to be allocated for individual and group advisement in order to create a sense of belonging and to assure that the necessary information is available to all students.

Finally, the student services planning should include the consideration of possible job placement opportunities for graduating students. Not all enrollees completing the program of instruction will expect to secure employment in community agencies upon graduation; however, many will anticipate this outcome. Since the field of aging has acquired the reputation of being an employment growth area with extensive potential, many people are drawn to academic programs by expected employment opportunities. In order to assure that this expectation is met, time and effort on the part of faculty or staff must be devoted to the job placement process. There is not a clear job market in the field of gerontology at the present time. Some of the professionals in the field are employed in agencies that have "aging" or "elderly" in their title; most, however, do not. Therefore, it is usually necessary for the faculty member or advisor to help graduating students identify the employment possibilities and assess the potential of each opportunity. This process requires not only time but the expertise that results from extensive faculty-community contacts as well. Often the field placement coordinator carries this responsibility since that individual is most familiar with many of the local community agencies. The planning for staff time and involvement in job placement should assure that the final result of the educational program—jobs—will really occur.

## Stage Eight: Staffing and Organizational Structure

By the completion of the program planning for course work, field placement, and student services, staffing requirements should have become quite obvious. There will be needs for instructors in several areas, some recruited from within the institution, others employed from outside. Directors of several established gerontology programs have recommended that the best method of staff selection is the identification of existing faculty from the institution who represent related fields and who have an interest in aging. By assisting these faculty to build upon this interest, they then gain the expertise needed to teach one or more courses. In a time of staff retrenchment such as the present, this is probably an approach that would be well received by many faculty members and would be accorded strong endorsement from institution administrators concerned about faculty workload distribution.

On the other hand, it is possible to recruit new faculty with extensive academic and community experience in the field of aging. A growing number of high-quality doctoral programs offer gerontology instruction in connection with a traditional disciplinary program of studies, and graduates are becoming increasingly available. This staffing approach will increase the necessity of new financial resources, but it also immediately involves some faculty who are knowledgeable and visible in the field of gerontology. These faculty can act as internal catalysts for the program and can help to socialize both students and retrained faculty.

Another staffing decision required early in the evolution of a gerontology education program relates to the process of initiating the instructional program. If existing faculty are to be included, they may need several months to gain familiarity with the field of gerontology and to plan the courses they expect to teach. Often existing faculty are given a reduced teaching load for a semester in order to assure that new course preparation is accomplished. This means that startup time may be extended and actual program initiation postponed for a semester to a year. This delay may prove beneficial, for it allows time for faculty interaction and increased communication as well as for expanded knowledge about each other, the program, and the community service system in aging.

A longer developmental period also allows for the formation of advisory committees from the university and the community. Since faculty members from several departments within the institution have potential input to offer, an advisory committee is often formed to represent all of the interested fields. This can aid in coordination, communication, and the institutional political support base for the emerging program. Similarly, an advisory body from the community may prove helpful. The composition of this group could include representatives of senior citizen groups, service agencies, and governmental units. These community advisory groups often have substantial interest in the development of a gerontology education program since it may affect their constituencies, provide career development opportunities for agency staff members, and represent a substantial resource for program evaluation and improvement.

In addition to the faculty and course development planning process, it is imperative at this juncture for the initial decision to be made on the organizational structure for the gerontology education program. Whether the unit will be a department, center, interdepartmental committee, or intradepartmental unit will be primarily determined in some of the earlier stages of program development. However, questions will still remain regarding the authority of the unit in relation to the institution as a whole, the number and type of administrators and support staff needed, the placement of the unit within the institutional organizational structure, and the internal governance structure (e.g., curriculum and personnel committees). Some of these decisions on internal organization may be made during the initial operationalization of the program, but it is helpful to clarify as many of the parameters as possible in order for staff and faculty to concentrate on program outcomes rather than on internal process development during the first year of program operation.

## Stage Nine: Assessment of Required Resources

Any new program of instruction is likely to require resources exceeding the typical operating expenses generally allocated to ongoing programs. Although it is currently popular to suggest that by reallocating staff and operating funds, new activities can be initiated without incurring major increases in costs, this is usually not the case. The required resources are generally of three types: money, community assistance, and personnel. The personnel requirements have been discussed as a part of stage eight, but it must be assumed that some additional funds will be required for the increased administration, field practica, faculty, and student services that will become a part of the new instructional program.

Financial resources are always a major concern for existing as well as new academic program units. Money may come from internal institutional sources, from in-kind contributions of faculty time or departmental administration, from government grants and contracts, or from private sources such as bequests and foundation gifts. The most coveted financial resources are those of the regular institutional budget. Often referred to as "hard dollars" since they are expected to continue into the future, institutional resources are difficult to acquire because of financial constraints and administrative reluctance to reallocate resources from traditional but declining academic units to those currently in vogue. There is, however, the recognition by many institutional leaders that gerontology represents a field with the ability to attract students and to assume an ongoing service within academe; therefore, some insightful administrators are assuring gerontology education the hard dollars necessary for security and survival.

In-kind contributions from faculty or departments are also a substantial and valued addition to any developing program. Since current faculty are being paid by some institutional unit, it may be possible to convince the faculty member's department chairperson that release time for gerontology instruction is appropriate. This would provide a means for a current faculty member to teach a course or two in gerontology without cost to the new program. Release faculty time is obviously very advantageous for the gerontology education unit; however, the difficulty comes at some point in the future when the other unit decides that it can no longer continue the contribution unless it receives something in return. One way of providing this tradeoff is to have the faculty member teach a gerontology course offered by his primary department rather than the gerontology unit. By this means, the student credit hour production will remain with the home department rather than gerontology, but the course will still be available to students needing it to fulfill gerontology program requirements.

Government funding is another source of financial support. This source has proven to be very popular during the past ten years and most of the current programs have received at least a portion of their financial resources from training or research grants. There are several federal sources of gerontology education funding at the present time. The Administration on Aging (AoA), in the Department of Health, Education and Welfare, currently provides funds for planning of gerontology education and for the operation of career training programs—primarily programs at the master's and baccalaureate levels focusing on professional outcomes. These programs are operated under Title IV-A of the Older Americans Act of 1965. The Administration on Aging also offers multidisciplinary center grants for institutions attempting to develop or operate a comprehensive program of research, service, and education (Title IV-E). Both of these programs provide support for faculty members, program administration, and student financial aid.

Training grants are also available from the National Institute of Mental Health, part of the National Institutes of Health (NIH). These grants typically support faculty and students in the field of social work, but many of them have included an emphasis on gerontology. The National Institute of Child Health and Human Development (part of NIH) awards center grants to institutions offering doctoral level instruction in the traditional disciplinary fields. These programs are oriented toward the preparation of teachers and researchers who will work in institutions of higher education and who wish to pursue a scientific approach to gerontology.

There are many other governmental programs related to the field of gerontology which include some funding for instructional program support—for example, the HUD 701 program, Title 1 of the Higher Education Act, the National Institute on Aging research program, and the Title XX (Social Security Act) training program. Although there is much interest and competition for federal training support, these resources are not an unmixed blessing. Since a majority of the grants from federal sources are for one or two years, some programs have been established and then discontinued or substantially reduced when the federal funding was eliminated. The federal or "soft" funds vary greatly from year to year and provide little stability for faculty and administrators of developing programs. Thus, most program developers have sought increasing amounts of institutional support rather than relying principally on federal funds for an extended period of time.

The fourth type of financial support has yet to be extensively tapped for gerontology education. These are funds from wealthy individuals and private foundations and are only now coming to the attention of gerontology education program planners. Gifts are often given because of a desire to help people, as a means of assisting an educational institution, and as a way to gain immortality through having a program or edifice bear the donor's name. Some foundations such as Kellogg, Andrus, and Scripps have provided funding for gerontologically related activities in higher education for some years. Other individuals and philanthropic groups are just beginning to consider the field of aging. A program planner would do well to explore with the institution's development office the plans for a gerontology education program; it is likely that this office will be more than willing to assist in the generation of additional funding. Private funding is especially useful since it is often undesignated and therefore can be applied to programmatic areas not covered by the typical categorical funds.

Another kind of resource needed in the development of any instructional program is community support. In order to assure the relevance of the instructional program, it is beneficial to have a cadre of persons from community agencies who are willing to provide guest lecturers to share personal and practical experiences. This also allows the instructor to introduce students to many local agencies as well as continue communication between the community services personnel and the institution of higher education. Community contacts may also be used in field surveys, practicum experiences, and job placement possibilities for graduates. It is advantageous to begin the development of these community relationships early in the program planning process to achieve some consensus on the development process and the intended program outcomes.

### Stage Ten: Timing Program Development Events

Although the planning process may well follow the stages identified, it is helpful to recognize that many steps may be delayed by deadlines or constraints established by other academic units or institutions. Planning will be facilitated if these delay points are identified and accommodated in preliminary planning. For example, the development of new courses typically requires review and comment at the departmental, college or division, and institutional levels. Approval may take several weeks to several months and the offering of courses prior to institutionwide acceptance is generally not allowed. Likewise the scheduling of courses may require substantial lead time. Class schedules are generally composed many months before the beginning of an academic term, thus causing additional delay.

Federal funding can also be a hindrance to prompt program initiation. Proposals for many educational grants are accepted only once a year, and the funding period begins in the summer or early fall. Program startup must be designed to coincide with these dates. Too often, a proposal is submitted, several months pass before a decision is made, and once the award is received, the funded activities must begin immediately. This sequence results in serious problems since it is not possible to be adequately prepared to begin a program on such short notice. Longer-range planning is also needed. Although much effort in the initial stages will be directed toward the implementation of the instruction, it is helpful to anticipate funding one, two, or three years in advance; to consider the expansion or revision of curriculum in one or two years; and to identify when in the future a comprehensive program review should be undertaken. This planning can help the faculty and administrator to look beyond the problems and pressures of the present to determine what long-term issues must be expected and addressed.

## Conclusion

The stages of program development for gerontology education are not substantially different from that of any other academic planning process. Each stage needs to be undertaken with as much involvement as possible from concerned constituencies: students, faculty, administration, and community. The process is somewhat more difficult than the normal academic program planning process, however, since there are so few generalized models in gerontology that can be easily replicated in most institutions. This lack of generalizability has occurred because the field is relatively new, because there is little consensus on appropriate goals and outcomes, and because the possible structures vary so greatly from one institution to another. Variance in goals, outcomes, structures, and programmatic emphases suggests that each institution must develop its unique activities with limited concern for the mechanics of other institutions. Thus, current gerontology education programs encompass great diversity, which is not considered detrimental at the present stage of development.

Two themes accompany contemporary program planning and development. The first is the need to achieve stability, security, and legitimacy. Most program directors strive to achieve the institutional support needed to provide a continuing funding base for program maintenance. This stable base is often facilitated by the establishment of a department and degree program in gerontology. Through the mechanism of institutionalization, it is possible to enroll many students who then will generate large quantities of student credit hours. The financial base and continuing institutional support is thereby assured.

The second theme that can be identified is the desire to maintain interdepartmental ties and community relations. Centers of gerontology which facilitate and coordinate interdepartmental activities are in vogue. Faculty can maintain ties with their primary department, a wide range of activities can be undertaken, and interdisciplinary courses can be offered. The organizational design and operating form to achieve a true interdisciplinary structure has yet to be implemented on many campuses, but the continuing desire exists to interrelate relevant departments and to make the importance of gerontology felt throughout the entire college or university.

These two themes are obviously contradictory. To gain legitimacy and stability, the gerontology education unit must become independent and autonomous; to gain an interdisciplinary structure, the unit must remain wedded to other departments and colleges. Thus, the program planner is faced with a dilemma. The question then becomes, Which is the best approach? Most gerontology program administrators find some middle ground which allows for both. This may be only a temporary phenomenon, for in the long run, each gerontology education program will need to either gain its independence or become closely and permanently allied with the traditional disciplines and professions.

# 11

# Models for Gerontology Instructional Programs

The several variables indigenous to determining and implementing gerontology education programs have been discussed in the preceding chapters. These include the issues, outcomes, administrative structures, credentials, curriculum, and the faculty decisions needed for initiating any program of instruction. Chapter 10 suggested a program planning process that might be undertaken during the formative stages of a new program or at the time an expansion of existing instructional activities is contemplated. None of these chapters, however, has attempted to integrate the numerous variables and decision steps into a comprehensive program model that could exemplify the key elements of an operational program. That is the purpose of this chapter—to illustrate the results of various decisions at the several planning stages so that selected possible gerontology programs are described. These models do not necessarily represent any specific college or university program but rather suggest some of the parameters that might be incorporated in an internally consistent and conceptually defensible program.

The preceding chapters have emphasized an analytical approach to gerontology education. On few occasions have the authors indicated their preference for one outcome rather than another. We have chosen to indicate the decisions and their implications rather than attempting to prescribe an "ideal" or "appropriate" gerontology instruction program. This chapter will deviate somewhat from this position. It is our purpose to provide four program models which are internally consistent, which represent appropriate outcomes at their various instructional levels, and which seem relevant to current societal needs. The models each have four distinguishing characteristics: level of instruction, organizational structures, curriculum objectives, and program outcomes. The models differ from each other in regard to the choices made on each of these variables. They would be presented in the following manner:

|  | Level | Structure | Objectives | Credential |
|---|---|---|---|---|
| Model One | Paraprofessional | Intradivision | Career/vocational | Certificate |
| Model Two | Bachelor's | Interdepartmental committee | Liberal education | Minor |
| Model Three | Master's | Department | Professional education | Degree |
| Model Four | Doctoral | Intradepartmental program | Scientific education | Concentration |

The four models are not in competition with each other. Each is offered to a different level of students and has its own values and defensible outcomes, based on a different set of expectations and purposes.

The models are the logical outcomes of the decision-making process suggested in the preceding chapter. Each of the characteristics of the models fits well with the other internal components. It should be kept in mind, however, that they may not be consistent with the internal dynamics of specific institutions. These models are based upon the assumption that the colleges or universities in which the programs are housed are typical in their goals and instructional purposes. Thus, the first model (paraprofessional) is appropriate for a community or junior college; the second model (bachelor's) for a liberal arts college; the third model (master's) for a college or university offering professional education; and the fourth model (doctoral) for a research-oriented university. In attempting to implement these in any particular institution, care should be taken to assure that the assumption on which the models are based is indeed accurate.

## Model One: Community or Junior College Instruction

Gerontology education at the community or junior college level is the most recently developed aging program in higher education. Although there are some programs that offer a liberal education approach culminating in an Associate of Arts degree, these are not common enough to be considered the major model for this level of higher education. These general education programs in gerontology are oriented either toward preparing students for transfer to baccalaureate granting institutions or for providing general education for persons wishing to pursue the study of the aging processes for its own sake.

The primary purpose of community or junior college programs in gerontology is the preparation of paraprofessionals and technicians for work in entry and semiskilled positions. These roles require some post-secondary training prior to employment, although many do not include the necessity for a degree.

The objectives for such a program would differ significantly from programs at other levels of higher education. Specifically, they would be designed to provide a general understanding of the basic concepts of gerontology and involve extensive opportunity for experiential learning in a job setting. For this model, the program of studies would not result in the award of an associate's degree but would culminate in the receipt of a certificate of completion. Course work would comprise only a portion of the entire curriculum; supervised field experience would constitute a major and integral part. Courses for this type of program would be highly structured and compatible with the particular occupation for which the training was geared. There would be few, if any, electives, and students would pursue a series of clearly defined and sequenced learning experiences.

The organizational structure for a program of this nature would place gerontology in a division with several related occupational units. This allows for the grouping of affiliated occupational programs so that administrative staff and costs can be kept to a minimum. The grouping of occupations within divisions does not suggest that there are necessarily courses common to all fields within a given unit; however, some common core courses might exist. Administration would be carried out by a faculty member within the division who, as a portion of his/her assignment, is responsible for program operation.

Faculty for community or junior college gerontology programs are typically part-time college employees, teaching one or two courses per year. They carry their faculty responsibilities in addition to being full-time employees of an agency that provides services to the elderly. This type of faculty assignment allows the college to utilize professionals who have firsthand, current experience in the field and make limited salary demands on the institution. Since courses are offered in a prearranged sequence, the staff understands the entire curriculum, thus allowing well-qualified faculty to teach several different courses at a given time and affording great scheduling flexibility, which permits the program to be responsive to enrollment fluctuations.

It is difficult to delineate a general program of studies for a certificate program in a community or junior college. Variations are practically as numerous as the programs themselves. Given the newness of the gerontology education programming at this level, no attempt will be made here to provide a generalized program. Instead, a model for gerontology technical training in the human services will be provided which can serve as a prototype for programs in related fields.

Two essential elements of vocational programs of this type warrant special consideration. First, they are not tied to the traditional time schedules found in higher education. The semester or quarter scheduling of courses is often dispensed with in order for students to pursue the course of study at a pace suitable to the content. Second, since experiential training is so important, cooperative work placements constitute a major part of the program. In a cooperative educational program of this type, the integration of classroom learning with off-campus employment becomes a principal goal. The success of a program of this nature depends greatly on the cooperation of employers and educators, working together to develop a comprehensive program of work and study.

A program in human services technology/gerontology might resemble the following:

*Cooperative Work Experience.* The student works in a position related to the occupational role he is studying concurrent with his pursuit of course work. The student spends approximately half the day on campus and half in the cooperative work assignment.

*Introduction to Gerontology.* This comprises an overview of the field of gerontology including demographic trends and the processes of aging from psychological and sociological viewpoints.

*Physiology of Aging.* This course covers the biological and physiological changes that occur with aging; it includes myths of aging, senility, sexuality, adjustment, learning, exercise, and related topics.

*Primary Needs of Older Persons.* An in-depth study of various needs of older people such as health, housing, income, interpersonal relations, and transportation.

*Institutional Care and Alternatives.* The types of institutions encountered by older people and the problems typically associated with them are reviewed. The course includes resident care and rights, rehabilitation, social living, psychological effects, and alternatives to institutionalization.

*Supportive Services for the Elderly.* This course examines community programs and services available to older persons; eligibility criteria and procedures are reviewed.

*Counseling for the Older Person.* This course is designed to provide an awareness of the interpersonal problems and abilities of the senior citizen. Direct contact with older individuals and small groups will be provided.

The outcomes for a community or junior college career/vocational training program in gerontology are best evaluated by the students' success in securing and retaining employment in the field associated with their training. If they secure jobs but do not stay with them, it would be an indication that they were improperly trained or that their job expectations were inappropriate. Both these outcomes, proper training and appropriate occupational role orientation, are essential to the success of this type of program.

## Model Two: Undergraduate Level Instruction

Undergraduate instruction in gerontology has expanded greatly in the past five to ten years. It is interesting to note that most institutions did not initiate their gerontology education at this level; rather it was introduced at the master's or doctoral level and has been extended into the baccalaureate curriculum during the 1970s. The purpose of this instruction is occasionally discussed in terms of preparation for employment in the community, but most of it is actually part of the typical liberal/general education emphasis that dominates undergraduate instruction. The goal of this education is a broad-based understanding of the processes of aging. This is achieved through a curriculum stressing the meaning of aging and its implications for individuals and society. Active intellectual curiosity, reflection and insightful collation of material, and verbal and written dialogue with colleagues are encouraged to prepare the student for a lifetime of educational development.

The objectives for the program are stated in terms of cognitive skills and emphasize the acquisition and integration of interdisciplinary knowledge regarding the role of the older person in the modern world. Although many objectives could be stated, generally students should be able to (1) identify and describe the interdependent processes of physical, psychological, and social aging; (2) analyze and evaluate the portrayal of older people in media; (3) trace the historical development of retirement and its effect on individual older people and society; (4) identify and describe their own attitudes toward and beliefs about the purpose of old age; and (5) select and integrate disparate literature into a comprehensive statement regarding the current state of gerontology knowledge.

For the undergraduate, a minor or specialization in gerontology appears to be the most appropriate credential. The academic minor allows the student to relate gerontology content to a variety of degree majors and provides maximum flexibility in course selection. The majority of the program would be left to the free choice of the student, with few prerequisites or required courses, so that the cumulative outcome would be representative of his/her interests. Courses could be offered on a multidisciplinary basis to afford the broadest possible selection.

An appropriate organizational structure for this model of gerontology education would be a multidisciplinary committee that would coordinate the offerings of the several academic departments. The committee would be composed of faculty members from several departments who would meet regularly to determine policy and who would teach the gerontology courses. No courses would be offered directly by the committee; rather, its function would be to monitor the departmental listings in order to assure a comprehensive instructional array. Individualization of the program would be assured by close working relationships between the faculty (committee members) and the students. The committee would have minimal staff, probably not more than a secretary. Its responsibilities would be carried out by individual faculty members acting as advisors or by the committee collectively. Thus, the committee would assure that sufficient courses are available, coordinate scheduling, and provide a forum for sharing faculty interests and resources.

In this type of program, since faculty remain members of traditional academic departments rather than having appointments in a gerontology unit, the courses are offered by the departments, from a departmental perspective, with little conscious consideration for the relationship among the courses. The integration of the various departmental perceptions may occur through an interdisciplinary seminar or through the students' ability to determine relationships among the individual courses.

With gerontology courses in several different departments, the strength of the minor will rest upon the extent of participation by the various faculties. Fortunately, if one department proves uncooperative, it is generally possible to convince a related department to step in. For instance, if the psychology department is unable or unwilling to offer a course on the psychological aspects of later life, it may be possible to have this content covered in courses in human development (home economics) or educational psychology (education). A well-rounded minor would probably include at least 18 semester hours of instruction. Some of the more typical courses would be the following:

*Life Span Development: Middle Age and Later Life*—3 hours credit. This course examines the normal development of the individual through the middle years and during the later periods of life. It includes units on personality development, intellectual capacity, adjustment, mental illness, and death.

*Social Gerontology*—3 hours credit. An overview of the manner in which society and older people mutually interact. The course includes content on retirement, social participation, social adjustment, economic considerations, and programs designed to assist the aged.

*Physical Aspects of Aging*—3 hours credit. The biological and physical processes of normal aging are reviewed. This includes the theories of aging, the normal changes that occur in later life, common disease states, and adaptations that can be made in dealing with older people.

*The Family in Later Life*—3 hours credit. An exploration of the relationships between the older person and the family. This will include family supports, grandparent roles, marital status, sexual relationships, and problems presented by dependent older people.

*Humanism and Aging*—3 hours credit. An interdepartmental approach to the aging process involving such humanistic disciplines as philosophy, ethics, religion, history, art, and literature. The course will focus on selected issues that affect the lives of older persons.

*Comparative Gerontology*—3 hours credit. This course will review the ways in which aging and older people are treated in other cultures. A cross-national, cross-cultural approach will be used to show the universal aspects of the aging processes.

*Geropsychology*—3 hours credit. An examination of the cognitive changes that occur in middle age and later life. The course examines recent research in the areas of intelligence, motivation, and learning. Students will be assisted in carrying out a small research project.

*Independent Studies in Gerontology*—1–6 hours credit. An independent study project designed by the student around his/her interests and needs in such areas as psychology, sociology, economics, or politics of aging. Literature review and field data collection are encouraged.

The outcomes of an undergraduate minor in gerontology can be measured in terms of student understanding and attitudes. Students completing this minor should have acquired a broad understanding of the many facets of aging. They should be able to read the survey and laboratory research with a reasonable amount of understanding; discuss articulately and intelligently the current condition of the older population; and formulate and defend the social and political policies that may need to be employed on the behalf of the elderly. Graduates should be familiar with the theoretical underpinnings of the field and be able to manipulate numerous concepts related to aging and older people. Enough thought-provoking discussions should have occurred so that the graduate can formulate a statement of the values and attitudes they hold toward older people and old age in general. These are liberal education outcomes—the development of a person who is at home in a variety of settings, who can encourage intellectual challenge, who has developed a conscious philosophy of life, and who has set a life course devoted to learning, reason, and humaneness.

## Model Three: Master's Level Instruction

Gerontology instruction in graduate schools has been primarily concentrated at the master's degree level. This has occurred for at least two basic reasons. First, many of the original program developers believed that gerontology could best be taught to students who had completed the general education requirements of the undergraduate level and who had a familiarity with the basic disciplines, such as biology, psychology, or sociology. Second, much early gerontology education was funded by federal agencies desiring to expand the availability of trained practitioners for community and institutional programs. This meant professional education, which has traditionally been undertaken at the master's level.

The third model to be presented, then, is gerontology education at the master's degree level, oriented toward professional service rather than a continuation of a liberal education or as a prelude to doctoral instruction in scientific gerontology. Most master's degree programs in gerontology are considered to be terminal rather than preparatory to additional degree work. Thus, Master of Gerontology,

Master of Science in Gerontology, or Master of Social Gerontology degrees have become more common on the educational scene, and such graduates are beginning to have impact on the service delivery systems of the nation. This third model program might be offered by a small university or by any institution of higher education with a number of graduate programs in professional areas like social work, counseling, public administration, human services, education, public health, home economics, or allied health.

The purpose of this professional master's degree program is to produce the motivated and skilled personnel needed to attack the numerous social and personal problems affecting older persons. This purpose intimately relates the educational institution to the needs of the community, state, and nation and encourages close and cooperative working relationships between the educational institution and the service community. Production of professionals is generally perceived to be a cost-effective undertaking—its indirect outcome being the improved quality of life for older citizens and a reorganization of community priorities leading to increased social justice—so support from state legislatures, federal agencies, and private foundations is typically available.

Professional degree programs emphasize the development of social consciousness, awareness of the community problems facing older people, and an activist stance toward solutions. The purpose of the instruction is not knowledge for its own sake, but knowledge that can be applied to the solution of contemporary social problems. This general orientation suggests that the world can be a better place if increased knowledge is applied in an effective and appropriate manner, educated professionals being effective agents for change. Vulnerable older people face such difficulties that only the federal government has sufficient resources and power to ameliorate the problems successfully. Thus, progress is most efficiently achieved through political means.

The objectives of a professional degree program are stated in terms of applied skills or knowledge which can be related to practice. These would include such statements as the graduates will (1) be able to identify and apply knowledge of the processes of human aging to individual older clients; (2) be skilled in assessing the needs of individuals and groups in the community and in planning actions to meet these needs; (3) have a high level of knowledge of self and the most effective approaches in using self to assist others; (4) be committed to working closely with clients without judging their actions or values; and (5) be able to describe and put into operation a service philosophy which will include optimism about the future, a concern for the welfare of the client, a commitment to service, and an awareness of the whole person. These objectives suggest some social values the student is expected to acquire and apply in the work setting. Basic among these is a commitment of service to others rather than motives involving self-aggrandizement or monetary gain.

The credential offered in this program would be the Master of Gerontology degree. This would require 30 to 36 hours of instruction beyond the baccalaureate, indicating that the student had mastered the necessary skills and knowledge to begin practice in an unsupervised setting. In many professions, the degree is the symbolic admission to the profession. This is not currently the case in gerontology since there are no licensing or certification requirements for practice. The degree can also serve to restrict the entrance of too many persons into the field. This regulative function is not currently operational since many institutions have developed degree programs without assessing the employment market for their graduates. It may be expected that increasing pressure for standards, accreditation, and licensing will lead to more restrictions on entrance to the field in the years ahead.

The organizational structure for a master's degree program often takes the form of a gerontology department. This is an independent unit typically headed by a chairperson who reports to the academic dean or the dean of a college of human service, public affairs, or social service. The faculty would have their primary academic appointments in the department, although many would probably choose to maintain ties with their department of origin through joint appointments. Previous community experience in service delivery or program administration would be an expectation for most faculty. There is an inclination for faculty to maintain close and cordial ties with the local professional community and to provide technical assistance and consultation on a regular basis to agencies and institutions requesting evaluations, staff upgrading, or management reviews. Thus, the structure emphasizes the establishment of gerontology as a separate field of education and reduces the interdepartmental cooperation evident in the previous model.

The curriculum is oriented toward the application of empirical knowledge to professional practice. This is generated by input from current professionals on the most important knowledge and skill areas and by a translation of recent research to effective practice. Instruction is not technically oriented; it is securely grounded with a conceptual framework that helps organize and structure the knowledge. The curriculum emphasizes administrative skills for use in community agencies; direct service skills for casework and advocate positions; and program development skills such as planning, community organization, and evaluation techniques. Each of these would be utilized in an internship or field placement of at least one semester in a community agency or institution where the students' activities and progress are carefully monitored. Whether this is undertaken by the community agency, the educational institution, or both, the fieldwork is understood to be an extremely valuable part of the total instructional program.

Much of the course work will be directed toward understanding the manner in which the community is organized to meet social and personal needs. Thus, human service agencies, public and private institutions, methods of securing government financial support, and assessment and evaluation techniques are important parts of the master's degree curriculum. Often this instruction is related to research on the effectiveness of current programs and attempts to design better service delivery systems. Understanding of the community is beneficial in identifying potential employment, so field visits and lectures by staff of community agencies are generally included in the course program.

As stated above, a master's degree curriculum would include 30 to 36 semester hours of course work, some of which might be taken outside the gerontology department. Courses would typically be sequentially arranged so an orderly development of content would be provided. A curriculum might include courses such as the following:

*Applied Social Gerontology*—3 hours credit. An introduction to the social changes that occur in later life and the ways in which our society has responded to the needs of an expanding older population. Emphasis will be placed on the local community and the services provided by institutions and agencies to older people.

*Applied Psychological Gerontology*—3 hours credit. An understanding of the psychological changes that typically occur in later life and the methods professionals can use in relating to older people. Emphasis will be placed on the development of techniques and skills for working effectively with various types of older persons.

*Programs and Services for the Aging*—3 hours credit. An historical survey of the development and effect of government programs for older people. The principles and philosophy of government involvement, the developmental stages of several contemporary programs, and the current trends in government support will be examined.

*Health Aspects of Aging*—3 hours credit. An overview of normal physical changes of later life and the ways in which these changes affect the vitality, mobility, energy, and general well-being of older people. Common diseases, treatment regimens, and health services will be included.

*Economics of Aging*—3 hours credit. An examination of the financial impact of an aging population on the nation. This will include costs of government programs, pensions, employment concerns, financial status of the elderly, and public policy implications of the increasing costs of supporting a large older population.

*Educational Gerontology*—3 hours credit. An introduction to the programs and potential of education for assisting the elderly. This would include the preparation and implementation of instruction for the elderly, public information and education about aging, and preparation of professionals for service to older citizens.

*Program Planning for the Elderly*—3 hours credit. An opportunity for the student to gain practical experience in designing community projects to assess needs and evaluate program outcomes. A major project will allow the testing of skills in the planning and developmental processes.

*Counseling the Aging*—3 hours credit. An application of basic counseling skills to work with the elderly. This will include observation of helping behavior, assessment of interpersonal relationships, practice in counseling settings, and group work with older people.

*Field Placement*—6 hours credit. A semester's placement in an agency or institution which has a substantial older clientele. This assignment involves an orientation to all aspects of the agency, a major project assigned to the student, and regular meetings with agency and university staff to evaluate progress and clarify understandings.

The outcomes of a master's degree in gerontology are generally stated in terms of skills that can be used to secure successively more challenging employment in a community agency or institution. The educational program socializes the student to the norms and values of the profession and enables him/her to identify closely with it. If the program achieves its goal, the student will successfully integrate his/her personal and professional life. There will develop a strong identification with helping others, with community concern and activity, with understanding agencies and government programs, and with a commitment to a lifetime of service. The profession will owe the graduate a living, but the graduate will owe the profession a life.

## Model Four: Doctoral Level Instruction

Doctoral level instruction was probably the earliest established approach to gerontology education. Because interest in the variable of age could be incorporated in the ongoing research of several disciplines, research training was able to develop with little notice, limited outside funding, and no additional faculty or staff resources. As awareness of the potential for research and teaching spread, a more formalized approach in several disciplines developed to prepare students at the doctoral level for careers in gerontology. These careers generally involve university or college teaching and have expanded rapidly with the growth of instructional programs.

The doctoral model of gerontology education does not culminate in a gerontology degree. Rather, at this level it is more appropriate and more common to develop a gerontology concentration within one of the disciplines. This does not require the establishment of new degree programs but does allow a new emphasis responsive to the changing social and academic scene. Persons completing the program typically receive a disciplinary Ph.D., which signifies the highest level of academic achievement, and a concentration in gerontology, which indicates special knowledge and skill in that area. Several years of study and "apprenticeship" are usually included in the program, which has minimal interdisciplinary cooperation and maximal depth and specificity in a narrow and delimited area.

The purpose of this program is to prepare highly educated and superbly skilled scientists who can extend the frontiers of knowledge in the quest to help mankind understand and control the natural and social world. The students and their professors are concerned almost exclusively with the generation, verification, and transmission of knowledge. They have limited involvement in its use or application. The assumption underlying their activity is that freedom from the bondage of ignorance will result in greater good and increased social well-being. Thus, the careful collection and organization of current knowledge, the development of methodologically defensible procedures for expanding that knowledge, and the discovery of new knowledge are of prime importance. Extensive training in research methodology and its application in laboratory and community settings are included as are the unique features of carrying out research on the older segment of the population.

Truth is the ultimate product. This is defined as ordering of empirical facts in a limited area of inquiry and taking the next steps in building a body of knowledge. Often this is accomplished by the development of a network among the researchers for sharing findings and insights, even though they may be in different universities, states, or nations. Thus, scientific gerontology education is a cosmopolitan undertaking that involves not only the resources of the single institution but a complex communication system involving faculty and students from around the world in a cooperative search for the truth.

The objectives of the scientific instructional program relate to the acquisition of knowledge and the perfection of methods to expand that knowledge. Student outcomes would include the ability to (1) identify and describe the major concepts, theories, and data available in the field; (2) describe the historical development of the field and apply its major principles to contemporary research situations; (3) observe skillfully and independently, collect data, test for validity and reliability, and analyze data leading to development of defensible conclusions; and (4) participate successfully in the reporting functions of research—paper presentation, report writing, and article production. These objectives all deal with the acquisition and expansion of knowledge rather than the application of that knowledge for the direct benefit of older people.

The typical credential of the doctoral education program is the Ph.D. Receipt of this degree indicates competence in the independent conduct of research and knowledge sufficient to teach others. The degree is usually accepted as the "union card" for employment in a university and often serves to legitimize one's existence for several years; after a time, however, other measures of productivity become more relevant. The degree program has traditionally been sufficiently rigorous to limit the number of graduates. This is no longer true, and many persons holding doctorates are forced to seek employment in areas where extensive knowledge is not needed. This is not the case for those who have a gerontology concentration. They are likely to have little difficulty with employment since higher education programs are still expanding. The doctoral degree remains the prerequisite for research and teaching positions and is likely to be so in the foreseeable future.

The organizational structure for this type of gerontology education would be an intradepartmental program, one that is totally subsumed within an existing department. Gerontology students in this arrangement are expected to meet all of the departmental requirements as well as the specific expectations in gerontology. A department that initiates a gerontology concentration is likely to be well established, having a reputation for producing quality graduates and research. It is probable that the faculty will come exclusively from that department and will have more interest in the discipline than in gerontology per se. They will have a lifelong commitment to research and will be nationally visible through publications and scientific meetings which report the latest in research findings. The department is likely to be quite dissimilar from an undergraduate teaching department. Faculty spend most of their time on research and publication while teaching only one or two courses a semester. When consulting is done, it is with government agencies, other research programs, or publications rather than directly with community agencies or older people.

Course work is not a high priority for students either. Although they take many classes in the doctoral program, graduation requirements are stated not in hours of course work to be completed but in the demonstration of competencies that display skills and knowledge. This is often accomplished through participation in faculty research projects as an assistant or apprentice. The curriculum, then, may be somewhat different than appears on paper, and many students discover that a two- or three-year program often requires four or five years to complete. The courses that might be included in a doctoral concentration within a department of psychology, for example, would probably include nine to 15 semester hours of work in addition to the other departmental requirements and might include the following:

*Human Behavior and Aging*—3 hours credit. An application of several personality theories to older people. The writings of Jung, Maslow, Freud, Erikson, and Adler are used to illustrate varying aspects of mature personality and explain the behavior of older persons.

*Intelligence and Aging*—3 hours credit. An analysis of research on the topic of intelligence and its measurement over the life span. Various IQ tests will be examined, and cross-sectional and longitudinal research findings will be compared in an attempt to understand the major variables in this area.

*Clinical Gerontology*—3 hours credit. An application of several diagnostic instruments to older persons. This experience will involve the student in observing, interviewing, and examining older persons in a field setting. Supervision will be provided by both the university and the clinical agency.

*Methodology and Aging*—3 hours credit. An examination of research adaptations that need to be made when age is a major variable in research studies. This includes consideration of historical contexts, cohort differences, instrumentality, motivation, timing, subject anxiety, and environmental setting.

*Independent Study in Gerontology*—3 hours credit. The development of a research project that can be undertaken in the laboratory or the community. The project should relate closely to the student's primary area of interest, be completed during one semester, and include collection of primary data.

The outcomes of a doctoral concentration in gerontology would include extensive knowledge in a narrowly defined area of inquiry, skill in research design and methodology, and socialization to the search for truth. A cosmopolitan approach reaching beyond the local institution allows the disciplinary researcher to share findings and insights with the national and international community of scholars in his/her field of interest. Through extensive preparation these graduates are able to provide the leadership within institutions of higher education for the development and expansion of gerontology education in the years ahead.

## Conclusions

The four models of gerontology education presented are typical of many programs that currently exist in American institutions of higher education. Although there probably is no program exactly replicating the models, there are many that offer a striking resemblance. However, many others have little similarity to any of those presented. This disparity is not viewed as particularly detrimental at this time. A process of winnowing is underway, and the most effective approaches are likely to emerge as dominant in the end. In the meantime, however, the models do offer at least four advantages to those who are seeking initial information on various types of gerontology instruction.

First, they are compatible with higher education thinking and emphasis. That is, the paraprofessional program emphasizes vocational goals, the common aim of community or junior colleges. The undergraduate program stresses liberal/general education, which is the traditional goal at this level. The master's program is oriented toward professional education, the most common instructional outcomes at this level. And the doctoral program maintains the commitment to disciplinary instruction at the Ph.D. level.

Second, the models are internally consistent. The interrelated decisions on breadth, separateness, and emphasis are appropriately made. Those that emphasize breadth (undergraduate) are oriented toward general understanding and do not attempt to include preparation for a specific occupational role or skill in a limited area. Those that involve depth do not claim comprehensiveness of philosophical and historical considerations but concentrate on one area of professional or scientific endeavor. The decisions are collectively supportable, and each model eliminates many of the possible and enticing alternatives.

Third, the models respond quantitatively to the needs of educated persons in the United States. At the undergraduate level, it would be possible to provide every undergraduate with an introduction to the field of gerontology. This is a valuable goal for an enlightened citizenry, resting upon knowledge of academic and humanitarian concerns. At the paraprofessional and master's level, far fewer persons would be educated, but they would have substantially greater skill than would the undergraduates. At the doctoral level, only a select few would be expected to complete the program and function as a cadre of future trainers and researchers for the field. Thus, the numbers of persons to be educated are appropriate to the needs of the community.

Finally, the models offer the possibility for involvement of many post-secondary institutions in gerontology education. Since undergraduate programs have the broadest mission, their development should be widely encouraged while a smaller number of paraprofessional, graduate, and doctoral institutions should be involved. Gerontology education can be designed so that many of the questions and concerns raised in other chapters can be answered in a clear and appropriate manner. Refinement of models such as these and application in specific institutional situations will continue to be necessary, but with careful planning, future programs can avoid many of the difficulties faced by their predecessors.

# 12

# Gerontology Education
# in the Future

Throughout the preceding chapters our comments have been restricted to contemporary activities and developments in higher education related to gerontology. It seems appropriate at this point to broaden our perspective and undertake some speculation about the future in order to suggest a few developments that may occur within the next 20 years or so. This type of star-gazing is laden with obstacles since no one can foresee future events with any real assurance. However, there are a few discernible trends which if extended could be used to provide some preliminary insight into the coming events. This chapter will attempt to describe these possible occurrences, first by examining national and higher education trends that will affect gerontology education and then by indicating some specific developments in our primary area of interest.

## America in the Future

The United States appears to be approaching a point at which there will occur a major realignment in our social structure; this adjustment will result in fundamental changes in the environment in which gerontology education is conducted. Historians suggest that there are watersheds in the history of this country every 30 to 50 years that alter the course of the succeeding decades. Many observers believe that we are nearing one of these intersections and that the next few years will witness a major change in American political philosophy. When this occurs, they suggest, there will be a basic redirection of the governmental and social forces, and we will be led into new and untested areas.

The contention is that there have been four primary change points in American history, dated approximately 1828, 1860, 1896, and 1932. These occasions have been marked by a war, depression, or election which redirected the course of events from that time onward. In each case, a new President was elected who chose to initiate a new policy, such as Franklin D. Roosevelt's decision to involve the federal government much more heavily in the economic situation during the Great Depression and in so doing modified the fabric of American society. These changes have not generally been accompanied by a revolution, but the resulting adjustments have been just as far-reaching and just as pervasive.

It is anticipated that another major change will occur during the next five to 20 years. It is likely to be preceded by a period of political instability, a breaking down of the traditional political alignments, and a crucial election that will provide a mandate for a new administration to initiate alternative directions in government and private policy. Although the expected change will doubtless have a strong economic basis, it can be anticipated to have a substantial effect on government involvement in social and health programs for the population generally and older people specifically. Thus, the resulting social arrangements are likely either to provide huge new infusions of government funds into programs designed to improve the quality of life and assure social justice, or to cause the government to withdraw from many of its commitments in the human services area and to allow the individual to become more responsible for his own welfare. Whichever way the movement occurs, it is likely that it will be reasonably abrupt and severe, leading to some dislocation during a time of readjustment.

Although it is probably premature to speculate on the direction of this anticipated change, the overwhelming passage of Proposition 13 in California (to limit the amount and increase of property taxes) during June of 1978 and similar movements in numerous other states suggest that the result may be reduced government spending, especially in areas generally considered to be unneeded or inefficient— social welfare, human services, and education. If this is the case, the rapid expansion of community programs for the elderly could cease and retrenchment might occur in the activities institutions of higher education have undertaken in this area. The "taxpayer revolt" may not materialize, but it certainly is developing a great deal of support at present and wary consideration should be accorded its impact on future developments. Extreme caution in program expansion should become evident, since financial support now considered "hard" may quickly become very "soft."

If, on the other hand, the change expands government involvement in the lives of its citizens, then aging programs and gerontology education would be in a magnificent position to benefit from the increased largess. However, this alternative should be viewed with caution also. There are those who suggest that we are currently delivering too many services with too little knowledge; that is, we are training persons for careers in the human and health services without clear data on which approaches are most likely to succeed and what knowledge is most valuable. If increased funds become available, the question should be raised as to whether we can utilize them well. Could we really double our training capacity without unconscionable waste and inefficiency? Can we afford to create new programs of study without experienced faculty? Can we hope to serve people well without better measures of need and outcome? Thus, the future may hold major changes for gerontology education. If the watershed does occur, we will need to be prepared for it, to be expecting its ramifications, and to have contingency plans for its likely eventualities.

## Higher Education in the Future

Institutions of higher education will also face serious challenges in the coming years. In addition to responding to the changes occurring in the larger society, they may be expected to experience a critical reevaluation of their role and function, as taxpayers and other constituents seek to determine the efficiency and effectiveness of their instructional programs. Concomitant with this outside scrutiny, colleges and universities will discover their own aging as faculties become older, tenure densities increase, and alternatives to regular faculty become increasingly common. This movement signals the end of the growth period for higher education and the onset of a time of stability, limited growth, and retrenchment. Although nontraditional students and processes will be employed, there is little likelihood of a return to the golden age of the 1950s. Higher education in the next decade or two will be an organization seeking progress in terms of quality and not of growth. It will be a difficult and trying time for all but the most well-endowed and prestigious institutions.

*A more open system.*  Higher education has always maintained a balance between responsiveness to the larger society and separateness from the antics of the real world. As molders of the culture and its outspoken critics, faculty members at many traditional institutions have sought to remain aloof from the political and social struggles of the day. Some of the newer institutions, especially the community and junior colleges, have established closer ties to local constituencies while attempting to maintain minimal independence from the political and power structures of their communities. The ability to maintain autonomy, however, is now very tenuous, and all levels of institutions are being forced (or are choosing) to accept more direction and control from groups and individuals outside the education establishment.

Although some institutions may attempt to ignore the claims of constituent groups, most will find it necessary to develop greater openness in the decision process and to adhere more closely to the new expectations. Governing boards, parents, students, benefactors, ethnic groups, legislatures, businesses, federal agencies, and taxpayers are each placing demands and restrictions on educational institutions and expecting continually greater responsiveness than in the past. This development is clearly seen in two parallel developments, decline of faculty control and accountability.

Faculty historically have been the source of authority in institutions of higher education. In contemporary times, they have held the ultimate power, and a vote of no confidence by this group was tantamount to termination of any administrator. However, faculty authority is difficult to organize and slow to respond, so in a dynamic state such as we find today, faculty control is being steadily eroded by centralization, bureaucratization, and administration. Centralization of authority has been caused by legislatures, taxpayers, and governing boards who demand greater accountability and coordination of higher education. This trend has resulted in the establishment of state coordinating councils, consolidation of public institutions into larger systems, and the development of consortia in which smaller institutions can effectively utilize scarce resources through cooperative endeavors. The resulting complexity has caused the expansion of the number and type of administrators needed to maintain the systems. Several new levels of line and staff personnel generate and report the voluminous data required by accreditation groups, coordinating councils, and the federal agencies implementing health, safety, and equal employment legislation. The administration has become overly bureaucratized as numerous committees and offices review and monitor program progress. This complex and changing situation has meant that faculty members can no longer remain current with legal affairs, government regulations, community demands, and local power struggles, so the leadership falls to the full-time personnel prepared to respond to outside demands—the administrators.

Accountability is another result of the expanding demands being placed on higher education institutions. This typically takes the form of increased pressure to specify the objectives of the instructional programs and to quantify the results. Many outside academe consider the faculty to be lazy, the system to be riddled with incompetents, and the graduates to be ill-prepared for life and work. These critics assume that programs should be judged by the jobs graduates acquire. Economic productivity is perceived to be the major result of a college education, and if this expectation is not met, then the education was pointless. Until more graduates are securely employed, we can expect major criticism of the institution and demands that the course programs become more relevant to the real and perceived job market. This will cause a continuing dialogue regarding the best and most effective education, with institutions of higher education being on the defensive until they are able to articulate more clearly their anticipated results in ways that can be understood and accepted by laymen generally.

*Graying of higher education.*   Universities and colleges, like the society in which they exist, are beginning to experience the results of an aging world. Nationally we are witnessing an increase in the median age of the population and a continuing growth in the number and percentage of persons who are in the retirement years. Although dire predictions of our nation's inability to care for its aged abound, these prognostications have generally been ignored by the citizenry, who have chosen to assume that America can solve any problem with additional federal programs. Since lobbyists for older persons' groups are the primary communicators of the aging message, their motives and constituency often lead the rest of society to believe that their concerns are exaggerated and occasionally self-serving.

The institutions of higher education, however, are now experiencing several attributes of this aging phenomenon. The mean age of faculty and staff continues to rise and professional mobility among institutions is rapidly diminishing. Tenure density increases and the imminent demise of mandatory retirement may prove to severely reduce the number of positions open to young faculty. Collectively these developments may be called the graying of higher education and may be anticipated to increasingly affect the functions of the institutions in the years ahead.

Reduction in the growth of students and financial support has meant that new faculty positions are not being created as rapidly as in the past. The oversupply of Ph.D.s in many fields is well recognized; an accompanying result is that current faculty are not able to relocate as frequently as they did in the past. At one time, the professoriate was considered practically a nomadic existence as rising and established faculty members could continue their climb to the heights of academe by changing institutions every few years in order to increase salaries, gain promotions, and acquire other professional accommodations. That is no longer the case. Although some movement continues, it has substantially declined, and faculty are increasingly realizing that upward mobility must occur within the institution and not by transfers among institutions. This progressively stable faculty results in a rise in the tenure density as many older institutions reach positions in which 70, 80, or 90 percent of their faculty have achieved this attribute.

The elimination of mandatory retirement after 1982 will accentuate this development. Assuming continued inflation, many faculty will likely judge their retirement finances to be insufficient and choose to teach some additional years before retiring. This will certainly benefit their retirement situation but will further retard the availability of positions for new faculty, will maintain a higher tenure density, and will leave the institution with a high salaried person rather than one at a junior level.

Added to this situation is the concern that many of the now localized faculty will have their expertise in areas of reduced demand. Thus, institutions will increasingly have high salaried, tenured professors with few students to teach and no personal incentive to retire or move to other institutions. This condition will probably result in attempts to retrain them for involvement in the newer areas of increasing student demand which seem to hold greater promise in the future. Retraining, then, will likely become common as faculty from the humanities, languages, and other depressed areas seek to gain knowledge and skills in alternative areas of research and teaching.

New faculty who do acquire a job are also likely to find institutions different from their expectations. Many financially pressed institutions are turning more to part-time faculty who can be paid less, are not tenure-eligible, and make many fewer demands on the institution. These part-time persons may be good teachers, but they are not likely to provide the leadership departments and colleges will need; they are likely to be considered, and to act like, peripheral personnel. Other faculty, who do secure full-time positions, are likely to be second-class citizens also. They will discover that they are hired as teachers without the titles or rights of regular faculty. They are not on tenure-eligible lines and often are accorded the title of lecturer or adjunct faculty. Although this type of appointment has been previously used for grant or contract faculty, now many regular instructors may be terminated on short notice and accrue few rights even after several years of employment.

*The limits of growth.* The previous sections of this chapter clearly foreshadow the expectation that the growth of institutions of higher education will cease in the future. With a decline in the birth rate and a reduced number of persons in the traditional college-age population, colleges and universities have realized for several years that the number of students will decline. This reduction, however, comes at the time when legislatures, benefactors, and community groups are recognizing how expensive higher education is and are demanding more efficiency and productivity for their money.

In the past, success was measured by largeness, and if an institution was not yet large, by its growth. In the future, a clear modification of this position is likely to occur in which bigger is not defined as better. The expectation is that both funds and students for higher education will grow much more slowly if at all, that more limited and defined goals will need to be set, and that program retrenchment will affect most institutions.

During the period from 1957 to 1967, financial resources for institutions of higher education increased at a rapid rate. The large population of college-age students, the general state of the economy, and the Sputnik-generated demand for better education aided administrators and faculty in securing increased resources from the funders of higher education. By the end of the 1960s, however, this situation had begun to change. The economic climate was no longer supportive and many states began to feel the squeeze of reduced tax revenue. Federal funding was no longer directed toward academic excellence but rather toward aid to minority and underserved groups. Thus, the expansion era of the sixties ended quite abruptly and without sufficient warning for many institutions.

Instructional programs, especially those initiated by federal monies, found their situation to be extremely precarious. They pleaded for institutional support, but many of the innovative and creative attempts to modernize higher education fell victim to the budget reductions. Program retrenchment became the order of the day. Student credit hour production assumed increased importance as budgets came to be allocated on the number of enrollments rather than by some other measure of value. Business, human services, medicine, and dentistry prospered, but several of the more traditional and less applied areas suffered by comparison. Thus, the reduction of students and budgets had led to reallocation of institutional resources and to a changed orientation of colleges and universities to the future. No longer are institutions of higher education willing to address all of the needs of society; they are becoming consciously selective of their priorities and concentrating their limited resources in those academic, research, and service activities with the highest expectation of quality results and institutional visibility. Growth is no longer the measure of progress; quality appears to be a likely candidate for replacement.

*Nontraditional education.* As the traditional students of higher education (the 18- to 22-year-olds) have declined in numbers and sought alternative entries to the world of work, enrollment has become a major concern. Although dropping drastically at some of the smaller, newer, and less prestigious institutions, the head count at most colleges and universities has been maintained or increased modestly. We now have the prospect of negative growth in the decades ahead. Although some institutions have reacted by hiring increasing numbers of recruiters, others have sought to identify new groups of students to support expansion of the institution. These students include older persons, women, minority-group members, disadvantaged individuals, and persons seeking career changes. Their current commitments are such that they typically cannot accommodate the traditional classroom organization and so request modified instructional arrangements.

One of the nontraditional approaches to education has been to allow more individualized instruction and lower costs by teaching in more efficient ways. This has been undertaken in computer-assisted instruction, programmed learning, and self-instruction, as well as in alternative arrangements such as credit for work or life experience. Each of these methods has achieved some success and has been utilized in several locations. However, they have not proved to be a panacea. Costs are often not reduced if the instruction is done well, and many students have chosen to ignore these individualized learning opportunities for the security and familiarity of the classroom. This type of educational approach is likely to be explored and advocated in the future, but it has yet to prove itself an answer for the difficulties resulting from declining enrollments.

A second approach has been to recruit a different kind of student, one who has traditionally not participated in higher education but who has academic potential. To a large extent this attempt has been successful, as attested by the rising median age of the student body and the number of women and minority-group members currently enrolled. However, many of these students have not been able to pay their own expenses and financial aid has been provided by the federal government in special incentive programs. So long as this aid is available, these groups will continue to provide a source of students, but they may be expected to decline precipitously if the aid is eliminated.

Third, there is a tendency to modify the traditional scheduling and location of courses in order to accommodate persons already employed who may be seeking to enroll in order to update their skills. Courses scheduled during noon hours, late afternoons, evenings, and weekends are becoming common so employees can pursue degree work while continuing with their jobs. This development is especially relevant for professionally oriented programs and may offer a means for recruiting students who would be eliminated from the traditional program. These students are likely to expect instruction directly relevant to their current needs and will advocate training rather than general education. However, this is a major source of students, and if their wants can be balanced with program emphases, an effective aid to both the student and the institution will result.

Institutions of higher education, then, are likely to be forced into major modifications in the future. With a smaller number of students they must seek aid from community and political constituencies that are likely to require adjustment to the values of the society away from the values of the institution. This adjustment may be seen in the increasing centralization of administrative authority, a growth in bureaucratic structures, and attempts to increase the effectiveness and accountability of the institution.

## Trends in Gerontology Education

The expected societal and higher education changes suggested in the preceding sections constitute the backdrop for continued development of gerontology education in the years ahead. As previously indicated, recent history has witnessed the rapid and somewhat un-

disciplined expansion of gerontology workshops, courses, and programs of instruction. It is our expectation that this pattern of
profligate growth will not continue but will stabilize as financial
resources become increasingly constrained and greater concern is
directed toward the improved quality of instructional programs. Although some new programs will be initiated, they will be the exceptions as current and future undertakings respond to the pressures for
increased conformity to some generally accepted standards for curricula and faculty.

In the future, these standards will need to be supported by
better data on the outcomes of various types and levels of instruction.
By defining the objectives of the programs in measurable ways, it will
be possible to assess the change that occurs in students' knowledge
and skill and to compare the level of preparation with requirements
for professional and scientific employment. This support and ratio-
nalization of gerontology education will be especially pronounced in
instruction designed for currently employed professionals. These
workshops and training sessions may be expected to emphasize the
useful and applied; this will force the faculty to design instruction to
be relevant to the needs of the student and practitioner. Thus, in the
future we can expect a clearer division between professionally oriented and academic or scientific programs. In order to clarify these
anticipated developments, four areas will be explored: the establishment of a common field of gerontology, the ending of program proliferation, the expansion of other gerontologically related activities,
and the next steps in the development of the field.

*A common field of gerontology.* Social and academic interest in
older people and the processes of aging will no doubt continue in the
future. As the number and visibility of older people increases, concerns of social planners, human service providers, politicians, families, and medical practitioners will be directed toward the needs of
this potentially vulnerable group. Likewise, scientists and scholars
will continue to explore and debate the processes and implications
of aging in the individual and society. These parallel developments
will culminate in a general social awareness of the condition of the
older population and lead to expanded activities in colleges and
universities designed to understand and ameliorate the decrements
of later life. More research will be undertaken, more teaching initiated, and more direct services to groups and individuals provided.
However, this does not necessarily mean that major new institutes
or centers of gerontology will be established; it does not mean that

degree granting departments will be established in most institutions of higher education; nor does it mean that vast numbers of students will be prepared for work in agencies serving older people.

Rather, we would expect that gerontology will become largely integrated into the common core of studies in institutions of higher education. Increasingly, there will occur an acceptance of gerontology as a legitimate part of the academic and scientific tradition, a part that can be communicated through various formats and alternative forums. For example, it can be expected that most psychology departments will offer at least one course in aging, and units of several other courses will incorporate some aspects of the processes of aging. Sociology, biology, philosophy, religion, and literature will do the same. Likewise, most of the professional schools, such as social work, adult education, public administration, allied health, counseling, and planning, will offer some orientation to the conditions of older clientele and provide a modest orientation to the accommodations a professional must make in order to deliver services to older people. Thus, the expansion of gerontology education is likely to occur in a decentralized manner with knowledge of the processes of aging being integrated into the general/liberal and professional curricula of the institution and available as an adjunct to established instructional programs.

In a sense, this will indicate a decision on the part of faculty and administrators to maintain gerontology as an interest area in relation to the disciplines and professions and to broaden the exposure to gerontology so that most graduating students will have gained some basic understanding of the area. Some persons would be specifically prepared for gerontology research or practice, but many hundreds or thousands would be sensitized to this area of knowledge and would become able to assume personal and citizen roles in more knowledgeable and effective ways than has been possible in the past. The major developments in gerontology education will come in decentralized program growth, generally without federal funding or major announcement of new instructional units. It will come quietly, a course or unit at a time; there will be no grand plan to promote the study of gerontology within institutions of higher education; rather, unnoticed incremental growth will involve increasing numbers of faculty and students in this area of knowledge.

*The end of program proliferation.* During the past five years there has been a major expansion in the number of degree and certificate programs in gerontology. These have occurred at all levels of higher education and have led to the establishment of new orga-

nizational units such as institutes, centers, and departments of gerontology. We believe that the bulk of this organizational growth has
been completed, that future developments will not include the creation of numerous new programs, but that the number of departments, centers, and institutes will stabilize in the next three to five
years and remain generally constant into the next century. This
belief derives from the predictions of retrenchment in higher education and of reduced federal support for preservice training. These
developments are expected to be major obstacles to the creation of
new degrees or organizational structures and will eventually lead to
the achievement of equilibrium between program productivity and
occupational opportunity. There will undoubtedly be minor adjustments as some levels (especially associate degree programs) are more
widely accepted and implemented, but the overall result will not be
major expansion.

Similar stability is likely to occur in the size of current programs.
Although the intent in the past has been to achieve continued
growth, many programs have already reached their optimum size
and are not likely to experience further expansion of staff or students.
Although liberal gerontology education is likely to develop as a major
market, this will be addressed through the traditional departments,
not independent gerontology units. Consequently, the units will deal
more with the preparation of professionals, for whom a limited market will be available. Thus, continued growth of gerontology organizational units is expected to occur in program quality rather than
in the size of staff or budget.

This movement will be buttressed by increasing attention being
devoted to the development and implementation of program standards for gerontology education. The rapid expansion of programs
and degrees has led several national leaders to suggest that both
students and employers need the protection that could be achieved
by the establishment of some type of academic standards. These,
they believe, will be necessary if the field is to gain and maintain
legitimacy in the professional area. Improved program quality will
result if standards can be established by the national or regional
associations. These criteria may involve faculty preparation, library
holdings, curricular coverage, or credit requirements. The form
these arrangements will take is not at all clear at the present time.
There are those who would like to encourage the establishment of
a full-fledged system of accreditation; others prefer the much more
informal approach of assisting developing programs so they might
profit from the experience of the more senior members of the field.

The Association for Gerontology in Higher Education and the Western Gerontological Society are both very active in this area. AGHE has initiated a project to generate some consensus within the field on standards, while Western has published a series of definitions designed to assure greater consistency in terminology among the current faculty and administrators. Although it is too early to speculate on the specific outcomes of these activities, it is reasonable to assume that some kind of national or regional statement on program criteria will occur in the next few years and that institutions will be expected to show that their faculty, curricula, structures, and outcomes meet the norms set collectively for all gerontology education programs.

*Expansion of gerontologically related activities.* Although distinguishable programs of gerontology instruction may not expand rapidly in the years ahead, neither should it be expected that colleges and universities will reduce their activities in this important area. Many institutions of higher education will choose to develop continuing education or community service activities rather than expand the credit instruction of the regular course program. This development may involve the establishment of new organizational units or the utilization of existing units for the delivery of services to older people, for continuing education of professionals, or for enlightenment of the general public. In each of these areas, the institutions of higher education can exhibit their interest in aging by mobilizing available resources to focus attention on the needs and potential of the later years.

One intriguing area for development is the mobilization of retired and older faculty members to serve the institution and the community. Implementation would involve offering noncredit courses and lectures by these distinguished persons. Other activities could involve the senior faculty in the development of resource materials, audiovisual presentations, case studies, work guides, measurement instruments, readers, public information, institutional research, and continued personal study or research. The opportunities for an interdisciplinary group of scholars are almost limitless.

A second anticipated activity is the expansion of housing and educational programs for older people on college campuses. Converted dormitories and new buildings are increasingly being diverted from young people to older learners who welcome the stimulation of the college environment rather than the peace and quiet of the retirement community. These programs will appeal to a modest number of older people but may prove to be of substantial benefit to colleges and universities with underutilized facilities and staff who could be of assistance to this new client group. Social and community services may also come from the institution of higher education. Increasingly, clinics, planning centers, and social service departments are offering direct services to older people in order to provide learning experiences for their students. With the large amount of federal support available, these activities have taken on major proportions in some areas. In Iowa, for instance, the state office of aging chose several community colleges to be the Area Agencies on Aging. Although initially envisioned as a modest undertaking, these programs now typically receive more than $1 million annually, a substantial sum for a small, rural community college.

In addition to these areas, it seems reasonable to expect extensive growth in the continuing education of professionals. A portion of this instruction will occur within the confines of the community agencies and institutions as they develop their own in-service training capabilities. Many of these agencies, however, seem willing to have colleges and universities provide this instruction if it can be delivered in a suitable manner. From the community agency's point of view, this means that the instruction must be practical and easily applied to the problems faced by its staff. This expectation of relevance may cause tensions between the agency staff and the institution of higher education. If a reasonable accommodation can be achieved, however, a major expansion in the involvement of educational institutions in this type of short-term training will occur. Thus, institutions of higher education may be expected to become increasingly involved in aging-related activities although not all of it could be considered to fall within the rubric of gerontology education.

*Next steps in gerontology education.*   Development of gerontology education to date has primarily involved the creation and expansion of programs and the search for stable financial support for these undertakings. This has resulted in rapid growth and some degree of permanence for many programs. It would appear that many programs are now able to consider the next step in program growth and institutionalization. This requires change not in size but in the conceptual and knowledge base on which organizational and instructional decisions are made. There needs to be clearer agreement about which knowledge is to be communicated, greater clarity about the skills to be developed, greater reliability of the job market that will receive the graduates, and greater assurance of the articulation between action research and social policy. These four items provide us with the developmental agenda for the next several years, and each will be discussed briefly.

A first step in the refinement of gerontology education will require educators to expand substantially the available data on instructional processes and outcomes. Although researchers and community practitioners have generated a large body of knowledge over the past 20 years, and the growth of this knowledge continues to expand rapidly, there is precious little research or conceptualization which can be used to guide the selection and organization of this knowledge for instructional purposes. The question of which knowledge to teach, and through what process, remains unanswered. Although writers of popular textbooks have made some choices of what to include and what to omit, their motives and criteria are at best obscure. In general, they attempt to include a representative overview of the knowledge in each area. This may provide adequate breadth and meet the criteria for liberal/general gerontology education, but not the depth needed for scientific or professional education. Since the number of available textbooks is limited, most instructors have been forced to select the one or two that appeal to them. The current expansion in available printed materials may begin to eliminate this problem, but there appears to be little systematic thought directed toward specifying the knowledge a professional gerontologist should have. Some theoretical orientations may be more useful than others; and some case studies may offer more benefit than general role playing. In order to gain a rationale for the type of instruction needed, much research and conceptualization should be directed toward these types of questions.

Thus, it seems necessary to predict that the future will see a major increase in the amount and quality of research designed to determine the outcomes of various types of gerontology instruction. At the present time we have practically no data to rely upon. Perhaps this lack of knowledge results from so few educators having become involved in the field of gerontology. While many of the other professional fields have been represented for many years, professional education, especially departments of higher education, have generally ignored this developing area and have not raised the questions necessary for formulating a firm conceptual position.

A second and parallel step in the development of the field will require specification of the skills professional and scientific gerontologists should be expected to acquire. While liberal/general gerontology may place few skill expectations on the student, scientific and professional instruction should include precise statements regarding the skills a graduate is expected to acquire. It is generally difficult to construct these statements with sufficient clarity to allow translation into outcomes that employers and graduates can consistently understand. The current lack of clarity may have occurred because of the inconsistent definitions of the term "gerontologist," but now is the time for some institutions and associations to specify concretely what their products are, so that realistic expectations can be widely disseminated.

A third step for gerontology educators will be to address the occupational roles students will assume after graduation. It is increasingly important for faculty and administrators to examine more carefully the occupational roles taken by program graduates. This will need to occur through careful classification of the skills and knowledge which agencies and institutions require and increased activity in specifying the employment roles to be filled by gerontology-oriented graduates. In some areas there are movements toward revising civil service requirements in order to specify gerontology education for certain positions. Other agencies are seeking to create positions that require a degree in gerontology. Too often, however, these initiatives originate with the community agencies or program graduates rather than being facilitated and supported by institutions of higher education. A discontinuity results when graduates holding degrees in gerontology lack skills or knowledge sought by community agencies. The characteristics of both scientific and professional gerontologists must be specified articulately to avoid such conflict.

Finally, gerontology education needs to design and conduct research that will document the impact of changed public policy and programs on the lives of older people. If we educate hundreds of professional and scientific gerontologists, we should have the means to show that their knowledge and skill are beneficial to the community at large and older people specifically. Research needs to be conceptualized and initiated indicating that their educated approach to problem solving will lead to superior results rather than simply to different problems. Gerontologists are needed; we all believe it; but we must also support our belief with data that demonstrate their long-term benefit to society. Until this has been done, we will be vulnerable to charges of self-interest and amateurism, rather than gaining acceptance for a field of study and practice that is of benefit to the older citizens of today and tomorrow.

# Index